CAREGIVER'S GUIDE
FOR CANADIANS

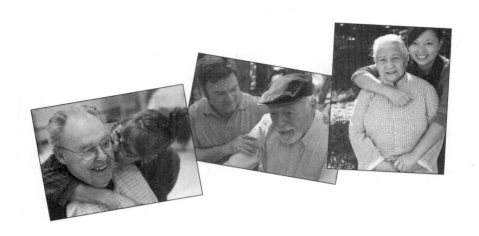

CAREGIVER'S GUIDE
FOR CANADIANS

Rick Lauber

Self-Counsel Press
(a division of)
International Self-Counsel Press Ltd.
USA   Canada

Self-Counsel Press acknowledges the financial support of the Government of Canada through the Canada Book Fund (CBF) for our publishing activities.

First edition: 2010; Reprinted: 2012
Second edition: 2014

Library and Archives Canada Cataloguing in Publication

Lauber, Rick
  Caregiver's guide for Canadians / Rick Lauber.

  ISBN 978-1-77040-188-4

Self-Counsel Press
(a division of)
International Self-Counsel Press Ltd.

Bellingham, WA	North Vancouver, BC
USA	BC

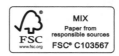

CONTENTS

NOTICE TO READERS

ACKNOWLEDGEMENTS

In memory of Mom and Dad.

With appreciation to Susan and Barb for their invaluable help with the "Aged Ps."

Thanks to Chris for her patience, support, and understanding while I wrote this book.

In recognition of all who selfishly provide formal or informal care, at any level.

PREFACE

My decision to write this book was prompted by a situation that is not going away — caregiving. Canada's population is rapidly aging, which means sons and daughters are scrambling to find and provide suitable care for their own parents. Unless these family members have been fortunate enough to work in the health-care field, they often lack the necessary skills, attitudes, and experience to adequately help.

There is a huge sense of responsibility, obligation, and even guilt for these adult children who may silently believe, "Mom and Dad cared for *me*; now it's *my* turn." In turning the tables, adult children do what they can but must frequently learn "on the job" while giving their parents the best possible quality of life. Commonly, family members serving as caregivers suffer from a sense of imbalance, stress, and myriad emotions that include anger, depression, confusion, and grief. This is certainly not the best for either the caregivers or the parents.

Whether you are becoming a caregiver, anticipate eventually taking on the role, or know of someone else providing parental care, you are likely entering into foreign territory. There is no road map or tour guide to steer you. As a caregiver, you will be called on to make difficult lifestyle, health-care, and financial decisions affecting your own parents. You will struggle and deliberate as to whether you made the right choice. Learn to accept your own decisions, your own shortcomings (you cannot do it all for your parent), and the crucial importance of personal respite (i.e., taking a personal break).

Trust me, this is not easy! I've walked in your shoes, serving as a caregiver not once, but twice — for both of my aging parents. My Mom had leukemia and my Dad had Alzheimer's disease. Through my experiences, I have gained a newfound respect for all of those working in care — specifically, for untrained family members (like me) who, often, have been thrust unknowingly into a caregiving role. I have also gained more respect for myself and know far better my own limits and strengths — as well as when it is necessary to take a break.

As you look ahead with uncertainty or trepidation, know that this is not a typical self-help book which simply aims to encourage or inspire you. The issues I speak of in this book are very real, and the tools and strategies I suggest can be very effective. I will share stories with you as to what caregiving mechanisms were helpful for me, and I will also discuss what was not helpful.

For the sake of conciseness, I have chosen to remember my Dad for the most part throughout. While my Mom's medical case certainly presented numerous challenges, my Dad simply outlived her and my caregiving responsibilities were extended. Not all of this may be exactly relevant to your own situation, but please glean what you can from it. It is my hope that when you have finished reading this book, you will have learned at least one new thing about what to expect or how to cope as a caregiver.

There are stories of confusion, worry, and neglect that surround the role of caregiving. These stories sadden me, but I would say too that caregiving is *not* all doom and gloom. While your parent's situation may seem bleak to you, there is joy to be found here — as you will see in the following pages.

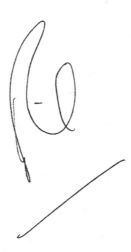

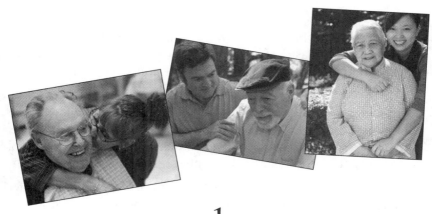

1
SHARING MY STORY

"We do not remember days; we remember moments. "

CESARE PAVESE

Most stories begin at the beginning, but for this story, it is more appropriate to begin at the end. It was June 20, 2004, and the last day I saw my father alive. This was a Sunday and one of my usual days to visit Dad who, at that time, had advanced Alzheimer's Disease (AD) and was living in a secured long-term care facility.

A "secured" facility is necessary for those with AD because they are prone to wandering away and getting lost easily. These facilities are not like jail cells; sunlight can stream in through large windows, budgies can chirp from a cage in a corner, and residents remain free to roam throughout the available space and are encouraged to do so. Elevators, however, can be security coded and exit doors can be camouflaged with painted wall murals. While you or I would be able to tap in a few digits or find the colourfully painted doorknob to easily exit the building, such restrictions can be enough to confuse an individual with AD.

The condition attacks the human brain and steals precious memories — careers, friends, and even family members are forgotten. In the early stages of Alzheimer's disease, a person can become increasingly absent-minded. Keys are misplaced more often, questions are repeatedly asked, and shopping lists become more relied on. During the middle and late stages of AD, a person can also forget the current day of the week, important news headlines from the past, and even his or her own birthday. My father, in the early stages of his disease, once overlooked my mother's birthday. Although I reminded him in time, he was quite distraught when he realized he'd forgotten.

Individuals with AD will also decline physically; too weak to stand, those stricken will often end up in wheelchairs. AD also affects a person's behaviours and speaking abilities. In my father's situation, he could eventually only mumble incoherently, if he spoke at all.

The aforementioned wandering also occurs in the mid-to-late stages of Alzheimer's disease. This could be due to individual restlessness, a desire to exercise, or a misunderstanding of the facts (e.g., a person with AD may believe that he or she can visit a long-time friend, when that friend has been dead for many years). Wandering, as an action, is harmless enough; however, when one lacks direction or cognitive abilities, it can become very dangerous. More than ever, local police detachments are frequently called by frenzied family members asking for help in finding a lost parent. More recently, Good Samaritans have begun stepping forward to help with locating missing relatives. It is alarming to think that a senior, wearing nothing but a nightgown, may escape from secured premises to be gone for days and at the mercy of weather conditions and other outdoor factors.

A further disturbing symptom associated with AD is "sundowning." This occurs between the mid-to-late stages of AD. The confused senior cannot distinguish between daytime and nighttime. This can cause havoc with his or her sleeping patterns. Should this senior be living with a spouse or family caregiver, there will be unpleasant spin-off effects: For instance, a wandering senior may keep others awake.

While many perceive AD and dementia as identical, Alzheimer's disease is, in fact, just one type of dementia. Other examples of dementia include vascular dementia and Pick's disease. Strokes can also cause dementia due to cognitive damage to the brain.

My ritual each Sunday included arriving at the facility and searching for Dad. He could be anywhere on the third floor — lounging in an armchair, sitting in the dining room, or sleeping in another resident's bed. The care staff on duty was always very helpful in locating him for me. Dad was a little unsteady on his feet and didn't even recognize me as his own son by that point, so there was precious little I could do with him. If he was sleeping, I would often let him sleep. It seemed frightfully selfish on my part to wake him up when he was obviously tired.

If Dad was awake, one of my favourite activities was to take his arm and walk with him. Dad had always enjoyed long walks and vigourous hikes so he always seemed more than willing to stroll up and down the extended hallways of the facility. On warmer summer days, I liked taking Dad outside in the facility's backyard. It wouldn't matter how many times we looped around the same sidewalk because it was always new territory for Dad.

In the winter, we remained inside the building and made for an odd couple — with me wearing my winter snow boots and Dad often shuffling along in his bedroom slippers. This sight always made the nurses smile and chuckle. When Dad was tired, I would read to him: Dad, a retired University English professor, loved the written word. In earlier years, Dad would commonly read some of his favourite titles to my siblings and I before bedtime. We were introduced to the likes of Mark Twain, Farley Mowat, Lewis Carroll, and Charles Dickens.

Now, I read to him — reintroducing him to the same authors he had once introduced to me. Given the choice, though, I would often choose to keep Dad moving rather than sitting idly on those Sundays.

Note that exercise is good for the body at any age. Without continued movement, the body will stiffen and weaken; older and brittle bones break more easily. When Dad was inactive, I was concerned he would not be as strong and flexible, or as able to heal or fight off infections.

My older sister and her two children would join Dad and I within an hour of my arrival. Together, we would have dinner. Our regular treat for Dad was to bring in take-out food; whether this was pizza or Chinese food, it provided a change from the standard nursing home menu.

June 20, 2004 was a double celebration because we were marking both Father's Day and Dad's 75th birthday. In his honour, we brought in seafood and chocolate cake — two of my father's favourites. Dad seemed to be in good spirits that night with a healthy appetite — he even drank a beer!

After the celebration we accompanied Dad back to his room. I hugged him goodbye — his somewhat musty, wool, button-up sweater tickled my face and Dad grunted his approval. How was I to know that this would be the last hug I would ever give to my father? If I had known, I would have squeezed him tighter and not released my grip as quickly.

My telephone rang at 9:00 p.m. the next evening. "Rick? This is Brenda at the Good Samaritan."

"Yes?" I replied, without giving the late hour much thought. "How can I help you?"

There was a slight pause before Brenda managed, "Your father has succumbed."

It was such a clinical term. Shock and grief overcame me. "Wh, wh, when? H, h, how?" I blurted out.

"Just a few moments ago. We were putting him to bed. It appears that he had a stroke."

The next few minutes of conversation were a blur; eventually, I remember hanging up the phone and calling my sister to share the news. She, too, was stunned. We had just seen Dad, alive and well, only 24 hours earlier.

My older sister and I raced over to the nursing home to tearfully say our goodbyes to Dad. He lay on his bed, half-covered by a sheet and shadowed by the darkened room. The only comfort was that he looked at peace. Brenda sympathized and explained that his passing was quick and without excessive pain. This seemed little reassurance, but what can one ever say at such times to ease the anguish?

Dad's body could not be stored at the care facility so we had to act immediately. With very heavy hearts, we called a local funeral home and arranged for Dad to be removed. I looked away as the attendants wheeled him to the elevator; all I heard was the clatter of the gurney wheels. When I heard the sound of the elevator doors closing, I turned and looked — but he was gone. After a few more sympathetic hugs from Brenda and her on-duty staff, we returned to my older sister's home and called our younger sister. As she lived in another city, she had not yet heard the tragic news.

The next week was filled with funeral arrangements, cleaning out Dad's room, and donating his clothes to a local charity. It all passed in what seemed like a second. Because Dad's room was immediately required by another waiting senior, we were obligated to move quickly. Looking back, I remember fiercely disliking having to return to Good Samaritan so promptly when the memories were so fresh; however, this was for the best. It can be better to face a challenge head-on than to deal with it later or stall indefinitely.

During these days, my eyes frequently welled up with tears. Little things upset me, such as spotting the bus I used to ride to visit Dad, dusting off the few parental mementos I had adopted, and even reading another vehicle's licence plate which began with the three letters "URN" (we had Dad cremated). I went for long walks without any destination in mind, just to escape the four walls of my apartment. I felt I had no further direction in my life. I functioned on autopilot through days and nights where I felt orphaned: I was now nobody's child.

I was not only a caregiver for Dad, but also for my mother. Mom was initially diagnosed with Parkinson's disease. This condition, a progressive neurological disorder of the central nervous system, can strike a young or an elderly person — Canadian actor Michael J. Fox was diagnosed with Parkinson's at the age of 30, while my mother was diagnosed when she was 68.

Parkinson's disease, for those unfamiliar with this condition, was first described in 1817 by Doctor James Parkinson, a British physician who published a paper on what he called the "shaking palsy." With this, Mom's hands would unexpectedly tremble; her handwriting became smaller and illegible. Her voice became a hushed whisper, and shoulder checking while driving became an unavailable option due to her more restricted mobility. There were many, *many* nervous moments when I was a passenger in her car.

There was medication, physiotherapy, and vocal exercises to help control the shaking and to make her life easier. There was nothing life-threatening; for Mom, always the stubborn one, Parkinson's disease proved to be an inconvenience more than anything else. I cannot say the same for what was to come next.

The far bigger blow for both Mom and my family was her leukemia. She and my father had both retired and relocated several years earlier to the warmer climes of Victoria, British Columbia, while the rest of the family remained in Alberta. Considering my parents' advanced ages, both were in prime physical condition at the time; I thought nothing of the possible future and the potential inconveniences associated with the distance between us. I realize now that this was a huge mistake. As a person ages, he or she will naturally decline so the person and his or her family must prepare. While on Vancouver Island, Mom and Dad did socialize; however, they built a very limited support circle so when all medical hell broke loose, my sisters and I had to act quickly. Although Dad had yet to be officially diagnosed with Alzheimer's disease, Mom's health news coupled with our joint concerns of how much we could help from a distance created an environment of worry.

There were few options. Mom and Dad agreed to return home to Alberta for a second opinion on Mom's medical condition. The diagnosis, little surprise, was exactly the same. While they were back home and temporarily rooming with my older sister and her family (certainly not an ideal situation), my sisters and I argued that we could provide far better care for Mom if she was situated locally. To strengthen our case, the three of us often spoke as a unified body — either meeting with Mom and Dad as a group or with the others echoing each of our messages.

Convincing Mom and Dad to move back to Alberta was a long shot. We were comparing the beauty and year-round warmth of their Vancouver Island home to short summers and bone-chilling winters. Maybe Mom and Dad still had a soft spot for their former home or perhaps they realized that their children were bringing up practical and reasonable points. In the end, my parents agreed to move back.

Despite that my parents were former residents of Alberta, they still had to apply for provincial health-care coverage. When my parents relocated from British Columbia to Alberta, they were covered by BC health care for three months from the date of their move. Upon the re-establishment of their residency in Alberta, the paperwork began. In the case of Alberta Health Care, applicants must submit photo identification (e.g., a driver's licence), a birth certificate or passport, and proof of residency (e.g., a pay stub or a utility bill). Despite being former residents of Alberta, my parents did not receive any preferential treatment; however, their former Alberta Health Care numbers were reactivated, making for at least one shortcut. In the case of other provinces, you should confirm the application process involved with your government health agency. For quicker service, I would recommend applying in person rather than by mail.

Initially, we found Mom and Dad a nice seniors' apartment, which offered somewhat independent living. There was a kitchen in each unit; however, most residents took advantage of the restaurant downstairs which served three nutritious meals daily. In addition, care staff could provide assistance with daily tasks such as doing laundry, providing medication reminders, or monitoring the residents' conditions. A doctor and registered nurse also made regular visits to residents.

Residents of the apartment building could come and go as they pleased. Visiting hours were unrestricted. A "great room" in the property offered space for residents to design different crafts, watch television, and play a game of eight-ball. Mom and Dad liked the building and got along well with their neighbours. My sisters and I appreciated the central and convenient location. I frequently stopped in on the way to or from work.

With Mom's leukemia, she required almost weekly blood transfusions at a local hospital. Occasionally, we could stretch these to biweekly appointments. Although these transfusions provided short-term results — I called them "bandage treatments" — it was a pleasure to see Mom return to her old sparkling self again, albeit briefly, where she had untold energy to tackle almost any job given to her. Even Mom, a dynamic woman and accomplished zoology professor who fixed her own bathroom plumbing and fought for women's rights, thought she was invincible after the process; she was found repeatedly climbing up the eight flights of stairs in her seniors' apartment building!

We became regulars at the local hospital. Mom always joked that she needed a "fill up" and that "the gas gauge was running low." Her lighthearted attitude helped to ease the strain of taking her in for what proved to become a full-day process. Mom had the easy job — she often dozed peacefully through the transfusions. As a spectator, though, watching the blood drip slowly from the bag above her hospital bed was painfully slow. There were only so many times I could read the daily newspaper, wander through the hospital hallways, or plug another few coins in the coffee vending machine down the hall.

Furthermore, coordinating these trips was no easy process considering Dad's declining condition. Eventually, we couldn't leave him at home to fend for himself for even a short period of time. Leaving a person with Alzheimer's disease alone can prove immensely risky because the person may turn on the stove and promptly forget about having done so, or wander away from home and become lost. Nor could we just explain to Dad that Mom needed to be taken to the hospital and we would have her returned within a few short hours — Dad would not understand or remember this. We could answer a question for him and he would ask the same question minutes later. With Dad being very devoted to Mom, it was even more likely that he might stray from home in hopes of finding her when she wasn't there. Eventually we either had to bring Dad along to remain at Mom's bedside, or otherwise occupy him during her treatments.

Fortunately, my sisters and I shared the workload. I feel that doing everything independently would have been far too time- and energy-consuming, at the very least. I recommend that you do whatever you can to distribute the work when it comes to caregiving — there is simply too much to do and too much for one individual to handle.

Caregiving can become overwhelming. An only child can be at a huge disadvantage without siblings to work with; he or she can, and should, partner with other individuals and caregiving corporations, many of which exist (you will find many links to Canadian organizations in the Resources section at the end of this book). Whether you are an only child or you have siblings, you should know that you do not have to look too far for support and encouragement. Take a few minutes to complete the Your Circle of Caregiving worksheet at the end of this book and you may be pleasantly surprised as to how many support individuals and mechanisms you can find.

My sisters and I often rotated responsibilities: One of us would chauffeur Mom to the hospital while another would engage Dad by taking him for a walk, treating him to coffee, or visiting the museum. Another process was to spell each other, meaning whoever was minding Dad would bring him to the hospital and trade responsibilities with whoever was with Mom. Sharing the workload seemed like the fair thing to do.

We also hired a private companion for Dad to accompany him on regular jaunts when we were not available. My sisters and I chose the private companion route for consistency more than anything else. A friendly face arriving on a regular basis can be comforting; the sight of an unfamiliar worker can be confusing. More and more professional caregiving companies are springing up; however, many of these companies cannot guarantee the same worker will visit each time.

To find our private help, we placed an advertisement in the local newspaper. There was no shortage of applicants. It was a matter of interviewing and selecting the best one. While past experience was preferred, we were more interested in finding someone with good character; we had to trust him or her to be gentle, understanding, and caring with Dad. Jannet, our unanimous choice, proved to be an absolute dream; she remained with us until Dad's death and even attended his funeral service. (See Chapter 8 for more information about interviewing caregivers.)

As Mom further weakened, she was admitted to the hospital. Although she was bedridden and the prognosis was not promising, my family still did not expect Mom's death on June 25, 2000. She was 73 years old.

While I had had grandparents die, those relatives were quite distant. I never really knew them, making those losses easier to bear. Mom's passing was the first death this close to me. Naturally, I felt saddened but I knew I had to carry on. There was little time to grieve because Dad still required attention.

Therefore, over the next four years, Dad became my primary focus. The property where Mom and Dad had been living somewhat independently was no longer suitable for Dad. He required far more attention than what could be provided. Missing that physical and emotional closeness he had had with my mother, Dad would "attach" himself to other residents. He would hover around them, rarely leave their side; obviously, his neighbours found this both uncomfortable and unnerving.

After some searching, we moved Dad from the apartment to another facility and, eventually, to a secured unit in long-term care. Along with moving Dad the first time, we moved my parents' Siamese cat. We had thought the cat could provide a sense of comfort, calm, and familiarity for Dad in his new home. Initially, the cat was welcomed; however, that welcome wore thin quickly when it was discovered the cat, when outside, could reach up and grab the home's door handle with his paws. The door would swing open and the cat would happily wander back inside. All fine and good, but the cat was not clever enough to remember to close the front door behind him! This posed a huge security risk to the residents, who may have unknowingly left the home themselves. Therefore, the cat had to go — immediately. Thankfully, my older sister adopted the cat.

When it came to the final move for Dad, we had little choice. He had outgrown the arms of Home Care (a government health program encompassing various services to help an individual remain living at home) and he had to be admitted into long-term care. Because of his situation, Dad was placed on a Priority List, meaning that he would be one of the first to be given an available bed. While we could specify preferred locations, this space could be anywhere and the family was obligated to take the first bed that became available. We were fortunate that a bed opened up at one of our top three care facility choices. There was no guarantee as to when or where the next bed would become available.

Transferring those with Alzheimer's disease is not always recommended because it can cause increased confusion and anxiety. The earlier move occurred when Dad was still somewhat aware of my mother's death; however, that memory slipped in and out. He would peer around corners and call my mother's name. He would regularly ask where Mom was and I would have to repeatedly remind him of the painful news. For Dad, there was no recollection of this so each report came as unheard previously — watching his pained response each time was heart wrenching. We could have easily told him that Mom was at a friend's, out for a walk, or reading at the library; however, it just didn't seem ethical to lie to him.

Perhaps the progression of the Alzheimer's disease was a blessing in disguise. As Dad's memory continued to slide, he, fortunately, no longer asked about his wife. He adjusted well to his new surroundings and seemed at ease. Conversely, AD can have negative effects where an individual can become angry and therefore potentially physically dangerous to those around him or her. However, Dad seemed relaxed and cooperative — quite possibly a testament to his character of being very quiet and unassuming. Knowing that Dad was comfortable and cared for by competent and professional health-care providers reduced my own anxiety levels; however, I always had plenty to do for Dad, whether this was paying the bills, chauffeuring Dad to doctor's appointments, picking up medications, or shopping for and delivering new clothes.

Balancing these extra duties, and often going steady from dawn to dusk, proved to be difficult. If I was not running another errand, my mind was always racing thinking about tomorrow's schedule or what Dad might need. Many nights I would fall exhausted into my bed and pray for sleep, but does one really ever sleep when in this role? I often wished for more than 24 hours in a day and even that may not have been enough time. Compromising on sleep was not the solution as it made me exhausted the next day. Every time someone brings something new into his or her life, it will demand a portion of their time. Caregiving did more than demand; it competed with my personal life, work, and outside activities. As a current or future caregiver, you can — and should — expect the same.

My employer was not the most understanding when it came to granting my increased time-off requests. It is my hope that employers, in the future, will adapt to allow staff more caregiving time to tend to the needs of parents. I, however, had to resort to other means to do what had to be done. As an example, I remember once bringing Dad along to my personal physiotherapy appointment. Dad, however, grew restless while sitting in the front waiting room and the clinic receptionist, unsure of what to do, led him back to my curtained-off area. When he saw me, Dad became more relaxed and sat while I was receiving treatment. Having my dad there, I could not physically and mentally rest to enjoy optimum benefits of the physiotherapy session, which was certainly not an ideal scenario.

Many times, I could not sleep because I was concerned for Dad. Insomnia was my worst enemy; this obviously affected my concentration and ability to function. At that time, I was both working and attending post-secondary schooling. Caregiving was done in conjunction with these other responsibilities and balancing the roles was challenging, to say the very least. If you remember nothing more from reading this book, remember to seek help when and where you need it before you burn out; a candle burning at both ends will, eventually, burn through.

Remember, also, to plan ahead. You pack a suitcase and map an itinerary before leaving on vacation; you make a list of required items before going to the grocery store; and you pull on your long underwear and boots before going outside in the winter — caregiving is no different. You must prepare. What will you do when your mom or dad ages? Aging is the natural course of life, yet so many adult children are ill-equipped for the consequences. While becoming a caregiver may not be an imminent consideration, it is a strong possibility in today's society. We age, meaning we physically and mentally decline. Never did this reality hit harder for me than when both my parents went through this process.

To their credit, both Mom and Dad worked hard and always provided for us; however, they fell short in providing emotional support or closeness. I cannot ever remember a good night hug or a kiss. My parents were not being mean or vindictive; this was just their way and what they had both been taught by their own parents. I now accept that they did the best they could with what they had both been given.

While I was never emotionally close to either of my parents, feeling like an orphan hit me hard. There was huge regret that I had not ever really known either of my parents. Granted, neither parent was the talkative type; however, why had I never asked them any questions about their lives? I know the basics such as their birthplaces, parents' names, fields of study, and so on. However, my knowledge of other personal information is very limited. Who were their role models? Did they ever do anything they regretted? What were their favourite colours? What were their memories of their own child-hoods and parents?

Over the past several years, anniversaries and holidays have dredged up painful memories. I wear a poppy on Remembrance Day in honour of our country's veterans; however, that flower is also a tribute to my father, who could not remember. While Christmas celebrations have changed over the years (and family traditions have had to be reworked), this festive season still reminds me of the past. I often wonder how society seems to focus on people feeling festive but how can people feel cheerful when they are not? The annual marking of Father's Day has also been complicated for me, for obvious reasons.

The old adage of "time heals all wounds" does ring true; however, one must be patient. I was told once that grieving is a personal process, so be tolerant of yourself and give yourself as much time as you need. If you know someone who is grieving, be supportive of him or her and remain understanding and patient. Show your love but give space; provide an empathetic ear but do not push him or her to talk. A person cannot, and should not, rush through, ignore, or dismiss sorrow.

In reading this book, you are taking an important first step as a caregiver, which is you are reaching out for help, support, and knowledge. You simply cannot do this alone. As a former caregiver, I can give you information. I intend to share what I have learned in hopes this may somehow help you. Through my sharing of personal anecdotes, I hope that you may somehow relate and learn.

Like so many other caregivers, the newfound responsibilities came as a surprise. Like a novice swimmer, I kicked and flailed but, somehow, managed to keep myself afloat. Although Mom and Dad had cared for me all of my life, I had never considered that the roles would switch and I would help care for them someday. Was this ig-norance on my part? Possibly.

During the course of my caregiving experience, my emotions ran the gamut. There were days I laughed. There were days I cried. There were days I was frustrated. There were days I was hurt. There were days I felt hopeless and completely lost. There were days I was emotionally numb and didn't know how or what to feel. You will likely experience similar emotions and many old memories will resurface as you proceed with your caregiving journey.

As a caregiver, I also became very aware of the struggles, the turmoil, and the careful balancing act required between living my own life and acting as a caregiver. I continued with my work, despite the fact that my effort and enthusiasm were dwindling. I ignored my friends not because I wanted to, but because I felt I had little time to socialize and my parents were my priority. I also pursued further post-secondary schooling (subconsciously, I must have realized doing this was important); however, I was having difficulty completing the homework assignments. Essays were being written at the eleventh hour and I did drop and postpone a few classes. As is common with caregivers, I put Mom and Dad's needs far ahead of my own. Like so many others, I was not fully prepared for this role.

Having twice walked miles in a caregiver's shoes, I feel well-able to share my experiences and knowledge in this book. I am neither a health-care professional nor a lawyer. Instead, I am a professional writer, a former caregiver, and my parents' son and, therefore, I am well qualified to share in these pages.

Through reading this book, you will learn what I had to learn. You will be better prepared to tackle and positively continue with your own caregiving role. While I have written this book in hopes of helping others manage and cope, I have also written this for somewhat selfish reasons — those being to help rid myself of those personal demons and my continued doubt from my time as a caregiver, wondering if I could have done or accomplished more.

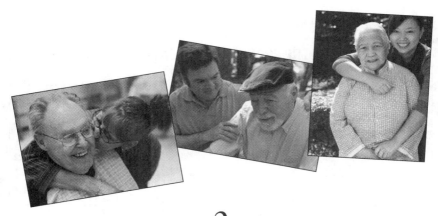

2
DEFINING CAREGIVING

*One person caring about another represents
life's greatest value.*

JIM ROHN

We are a greying population. The children of World War II's return-ing soldiers are growing older. These are our society's baby boomers. I fall into this category myself.

According to Statistics Canada's 2011 Census, the number of Canadians classified as seniors (aged 65 or older) is on the rise, with no signs of slowing down. Seniors made up 14.8 percent of the Ca-nadian population in 2011, up from 13.7 percent in 2006. If these percentages don't speak to you, another way to look at things is by total numbers: There are now nearly 5 million seniors living amongst us. Table 1 provides an excellent visual.

Table 2 shows an ongoing growth in the number of seniors for decades and illustrates why aging must become more of a national concern. In the past 90 years, this share of our country's total popu-lation has skyrocketed.

In looking ahead, there are no signs of relief. The number of Ca-nadian seniors is expected to nearly double by the year 2035, while our country's number of children will be proportionately reduced. As more seniors retire from the workforce, more companies will be losing the experienced and more knowledgeable employees. Those same seniors, now drawing public pensions, will impact Canada's

TABLE 1
PERCENTAGE OF THE POPULATION AGED 65 YEARS AND OLDER

Census Year	Canada	NF	PE	NS	NB	QC	ON	MB	SK	AB	BC	YT	NT	NU
	Percentage													
1956	7.7	6.0	10.4	8.5	7.8	5.7	8.4	9.0	8.9	7.2	10.8	4.9	2.6	...
1961	7.6	5.9	10.4	8.6	7.8	5.8	8.1	9.0	9.2	7.0	10.2	3.2	2.6	...
1966	7.7	5.9	10.8	8.9	8.2	6.1	8.2	9.2	9.3	7.1	9.5	3.6	2.7	...
1971	8.1	6.1	11.1	9.2	8.6	6.9	8.4	9.7	10.2	7.3	9.4	2.8	2.2	...
1976	8.7	6.6	11.2	9.7	9.0	7.7	8.9	10.4	11.1	7.5	9.8	2.9	2.7	...
1981	9.7	7.7	12.2	10.9	10.1	8.8	10.1	11.9	12.0	7.3	10.9	3.2	2.9	...
1986	10.7	8.8	12.7	11.9	11.1	10.0	10.9	12.6	12.7	8.1	12.1	3.7	2.8	...
1991	11.6	9.7	13.2	12.6	12.2	11.2	11.7	13.4	14.1	9.1	12.9	3.9	2.8	2.0
1996	12.2	10.8	13.0	13.1	12.6	12.1	12.4	13.7	14.7	9.9	12.8	4.4	3.0	2.1
2001	13.0	12.3	13.7	13.9	13.6	13.3	12.9	14.0	15.1	10.4	13.6	6.0	4.4	2.2
2006	13.7	13.9	14.9	15.1	14.7	14.3	13.6	14.1	15.4	10.7	14.6	7.5	4.8	2.7
2011	14.8	16.0	16.3	16.6	16.5	15.9	14.6	14.3	14.9	11.1	15.7	9.1	5.8	3.3

Source: Statistics Canada http://www12.statcan.gc.ca/census-recensement/2011/dp-pd/hlt-fst/as-sa/Pages/highlight.cfm?TabID=1&Lang=E&PRCode=01&Asc=0&OrderBy=1&Sex=1&View=1&tableID=22

TABLE 2
PERSONS AGED 65 YEARS AND OLDER IN THE CANADIAN POPULATION

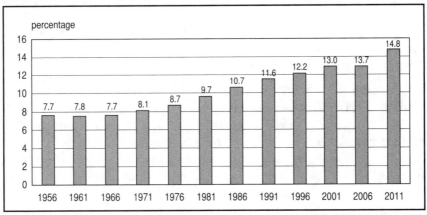

Source: Statistics Canada http://www12.statcan.gc.ca/census-recensement/2011/dp-pd/hlt-fst/as-sa/Pages/highlight.cfm?TabID=1&Lang=E&Asc=1&PRCode=01&OrderBy=999&Sex=1&View=1&tableID=21&queryID=1

economy. With increasing health concerns, which can come with aging, those same seniors will heavily impact our country's provincial health-insurance plans. Unless something changes, more family members will be called on to step in and serve as inexperienced and unqualified caregivers.

A high population of seniors is not just a Canadian concern; it is becoming a global concern. There have been reports of alarming spikes in other countries' senior populations. From 2001 to 2006, France saw a 16.2 percent increase in seniors, Germany experienced a 19.3 percent rise in this same demographic, and Japan reported a 20.8 percent growth. Should these numbers not speak to you, know that aging is a natural course of life and a high population of seniors is almost guaranteed as baby boomers age. This is an oncoming speeding car that cannot be avoided. With the rise in seniors expected, there will be a correlating rise in the number of professional and private caregivers.

1. UNDERSTANDING THE ROLES OF CAREGIVERS

A caregiver can be simply defined as anyone who formally or informally helps tend to the needs of others — mentally, physically, emotionally, or spiritually.

It's important to realize that caregivers exist on many different levels. There are the medical doctors who practice full time, the nurses who scurry from hospital room to hospital room, and the volunteers who push patients around in wheelchairs. A caregiver may also work part time and may not even identify himself or herself as someone caring for another. A neighbour could mow the lawn or shovel the walks for a housebound senior, a friend could drop in for a cup of coffee and chat, or a son or daughter could prepare and deliver a home-cooked meal. A minister can provide care and guidance on a spiritual level. A musician can visit a long-term care centre and entertain residents with songs. A small child can provide care by distracting a senior with innocent play. No matter what level a person serves as a caregiver, he or she is doing noble work.

Some caregivers are not even humans! A dog can provide care through unconditional love. Many long-term and acute-care facilities are increasingly offering pet therapy where animals either live in or are brought into the facility for residents. Stroking the fur of a dog or having a cat purr in a person's lap can be very soothing. Before you bring your pet into your parent's care facility, clear this with the appropriate authorities. Consider that the sudden excited barking of a dog could upset other residents, and the long hair of a cat could cause unpleasant and potentially dangerous allergic reactions for others.

We often think of parents providing care for their children. This is one of the most obvious examples of caregiving. With Canada's aging society, we are rethinking that norm and now understand and accept that adult children can so easily become caregivers for their own parents. Caregiving may inch up on you (e.g., a parent's chronic health condition) or it may happen overnight (e.g., a parent falls and becomes crippled). Should you become a caregiver for both of your parents, it can also happen both ways. You can never totally forecast the future. My father, on the one hand, was always a little forgetful, so Alzheimer's disease was not a total surprise. My mother's conditions, on the other hand, came without any warning.

No matter what type of health condition exists (e.g., cancer, multiple sclerosis, kidney disease), caregivers can face a steep learning curve to become more knowledgeable. They will research the condition to become familiar with the symptoms, outcomes, and possible treatments. Sometimes, family caregivers feel shame about having to care for their aging parents. Feared humiliation or a lack of understanding from others can lead to reluctant whispers of admission. This is unfortunate as caregivers should be very proud of their role.

2. REMEMBER TO TAKE CARE OF YOURSELF

Whether you are just starting your caregiving responsibilities or have been tending to your parent for some time, you will have likely recognized the incredible toll that caregiving can take on you.

One of the most common caregiver complaints is stress. Stress is your body's natural reaction to dangerous or uncomfortable situations. You can fight, or take flight. Any number of issues can be caused by excessive stress such as insomnia, moodiness, increased susceptibility to sickness, and poor appetite.

When my parents were alive, I found myself incessantly worrying about both of them, although their health conditions were far beyond my control. I am usually quite easygoing; however, I became prone to snapping at others. I also noticed that as I was rushing from one appointment to the next, I became much more aggressive behind the steering wheel. I paced impatiently while standing in lines. I repeatedly checked the clock or my watch while waiting at appointments. Many nights, I did not sleep well. My appetite decreased, and on the rare occasion when I was hungry, dinner was a frozen pizza, lunch the next day would be a leftover slice of that same pizza, and breakfast would be a cup of coffee and a stale blueberry muffin that I picked up on the way to work.

You must remember to eat healthily and try not to rely on stress or sleep medications. Maintain proper nutrition. Convenience foods can be prepared and eaten quickly, and seem like the perfect answer for busy caregivers, yet such prepackaged products are often full of unhealthy preservatives. If you think you have no time, prepare a number of slow-cooker meals and portion them into individual servings, then freeze them. Defrosting each meal in the microwave only takes a few minutes. Take a container of frozen stew with you to work in the morning — it will be thawed by lunch. Stock a bowl of fresh fruit on your kitchen counter. Keep your top desk drawer at work stocked with extra granola bars, cheese and crackers, or nuts for afternoon snacks. You could involve your family members with meal preparation, on a rotating basis.

When you eat dinner, make it a point to sit down at the table with someone else. Doing so will encourage you to slow down and converse with another person. Yes, I confess to having eaten out of the cooking pot. When eating, multitasking is not recommended. If you have children, you may well discourage them from playing at or straying from the table until they are finished eating, so why should it be any different for you? Help yourself relax and set a positive example for any children at the same time. Wait until you finish your meal before you make a phone call, concentrate on tomorrow's schedule, or read that doctor's report.

Before you rush out the door in the morning, ensure you eat something nourishing. Pour yourself a bowl of cereal, sprinkle some berries or nuts into yogurt, or spread peanut butter over toast. You'll find that doing this doesn't delay you excessively and you'll have far more energy to tackle the day ahead. In a pinch, grab a piece of fruit and tuck it into your jacket pocket for a snack later. Your body requires fuel to drive it.

Remaining hydrated is also important. Make sure you are drinking enough water for your weight and fitness level because it will help you stay hydrated and help reduce toxins inside your body. No matter whether you work in a high-rise office tower or in your home's second bedroom, one good recommendation is to keep a water bottle on your desk. On warmer days, drink more frequently to avoid dehydration. To help measure your intake, keep a large bottle of water in your refrigerator. Aim to drink all of it and refill the bottle on a daily basis.

Insomnia was a dreaded enemy for me and had obvious spinoff effects. I was exhausted the next day when I didn't, or couldn't, sleep restfully at night. Being tired greatly affected my concentration and performance levels with work and school. There were times I would have to ask for someone to repeat a question or thought, simply because I had missed it. While there are over-the-counter sleep aids available from your local pharmacy, consider other, more natural options before you begin relying on medication to soothe you to sleep.

Options that helped me sleep included avoiding eating half an hour to one hour prior to bedtime, using heavier curtains to darken my bedroom, and going to bed at the same time each night. I also experimented with a sleep hypnosis CD, which proved to be somewhat effective. You could also try turning down your heat or opening the window to allow your bedroom to become more chilled.

If you must have something to drink, avoid alcohol. Instead, sip a relaxing non-caffeinated herbal tea before turning in for the night. Try meditating or practicing yoga. While I briefly considered wearing earplugs to bed so as to block any outside noise and encourage me to doze, I realized that those earplugs could also block the ringing telephone, calling me to immediate duty. Move the television set out of your bedroom as well. Watching disturbing movies or news will not help you get a peaceful sleep.

You can also help yourself get much-needed rest by replacing an aging mattress or box spring. An effective mattress should be firm enough to provide support, yet still be comfortable. An older bed frame will also squeak whenever you move during the night, thus potentially keeping you awake. If cost is an issue, regularly flip your mattress over and invest in a good pillow.

Furthermore, when the human body is worn down, it becomes more prone to sickness. While I am no doctor, I fully recognize the importance of self-care for a caregiver and, even long after my parents are gone, I still preach this concept. It can be a very tired cliché, but it rings true nontheless: How can you care for someone else if you cannot care for yourself? I will repeat that continuously throughout this book. Nothing is more vital. When you are sick, you are little or absolutely no use to your loved one. In fact, when you are physically with your parents, you will pose a greater risk to them as germs may transfer.

Remember, your parents and their neighbours in care facilities are older and have weaker immune systems than you. If you are ill, it is not a time to be visiting. You will be more of a hindrance than a help. Quarantine yourself until you are better. If you must visit, wash your hands before and after you visit. You can also keep a bottle of hand sanitizer in your vehicle's glove compartment.

You may also feel depressed. This is a natural response, and you should not be ashamed of this. While a particular disease may be out of your complete scope of understanding, whatever you can do as a caregiver is very much appreciated. You are only human. As a caregiver, you cannot dart into the nearest telephone booth to change into your "superhuman" costume! With doing whatever you can, you are remaining realistic as well as helping both your loved one and the care staff involved.

Caregiving most often falls on the shoulders of a daughter. By their assumed nature, women are perceived to be more nurturing and make very good caregivers. Therefore, as a male, I was more of a rarity; but males are just as capable of providing care for a loved one. Thankfully, this understanding is becoming more socially acknowledged.

One must recognize and appreciate that the types and levels of care will differ between men and women. Celebrate these differences and allow for caregivers to function where they feel most comfortable. Men are equally able to serve as a guardian or trustee, to deliver a meal, to drive a senior to a medical appointment, or to accompany a loved one on a walk. Society has long portrayed the man as the strong provider; however, it is important to recognize that men have feelings too. While a man may hide his tears in public, he is equally able to cry. If you are a male caregiver, do not bottle up your emotions.

When I found myself bottling up my feelings, I compared myself to a pressure cooker — where the lid could pop off at any time without notice. In other words, bottling may lead a person to blow up in anger at the most inopportune moments and at someone who may not understand your situation. Find an outlet to reduce the stress. While I never found a support group strictly for male caregivers, I did ensure I found other means to relax. I shared with my sisters, I read, I went to the gym, and I went for long walks.

While caregiving is not all turmoil, you must find something that works for you as an escape. You cannot burn the candle at both ends for long before the candle burns through. Take some time for you and never feel guilty for doing so. This is far easier said than done; however, you will retain your own sanity and not become a martyr.

One of the best things you can do for yourself and for your loved one is to watch for your own signs of stress or other unusual reactions. Pay attention to your own body and note when someone remarks that you are acting out of the ordinary. Monitor these observations and record them on paper so you will not forget them. If things become unbearable, see your family doctor for a medical diagnosis. Take your notes with you so you will have something to refer to.

At the end of this book you will find a worksheet entitled Scheduling "Me" Time to help you make sure you take some time for yourself.

3. WHAT KIND OF CAREGIVER ARE YOU?

With the many unique situations and surrounding circumstances, I have yet to find a template that all caregivers could follow. Resources, such as this book, can only provide guidance; what your experience will become is yours and yours alone.

People vary considerably with personalities, abilities, mannerisms, and beliefs. What is "right" or proper for one person may not be for another. Different cultural practices may also come into play. Recognize your own strengths and limitations. The following are some of the questions you will need to consider:

- What can you do?
- How much can you do?
- Why are certain issues or projects important for you to manage?
- What do you want to do?
- How do you want to accomplish this?
- Who can help you?
- Can you work well with others or do you prefer to work independently?
- Can you lessen your load and delegate work to others?

It is perfectly natural to feel uncomfortable performing certain tasks. If you understand your caregiving style, you will be far better prepared to tackle every task that comes your way, and decide whether to leave it or delegate the task to someone else. You do not — and should not — always have to juggle everything yourself. How you approach your own caregiving role is always your own way so don't let anyone tell you what is best for you and your loved one. It's time to do an honest self-evaluation to identify your own caregiving characteristics. Good caregiving characteristics are described by Anne Togher in her informative article, "What is Your Caregiver Style?," published in October of 2009. (To read the article, search online using the title.) The following sections cover my experience on caregiving characteristics, which is a variation on Togher's caregiving characteristics.

You will likely recognize yourself as one, or a combination of, the following caregiving types. As you will see, there is no cookie-cutter caregiver. You may well identify with different character traits and not neatly slide into just one category. The trick is to know what you are best at and proceed accordingly.

At the end of this book you will find a Caregiving Self-Analysis worksheet to help you identify your strengths and weaknesses as a caregiver.

3.1 Independent caregiver

Are you determined, motivated, and stubborn? Do you want to tackle everything yourself? Do you feel resistance when it comes to sharing the work, or doubtful that anyone could exceed your own expectations? If so, you will likely want to do everything required by yourself.

So-called independent caregivers may feel, and appear, confident as they are handling the important affairs; however, they will be stretched to the limits and must become more flexible. Independent caregivers, more so than other types of caregivers, can be called on at a moment's notice.

3.2 Sharing caregiver

If you are able to collaborate, are able to balance the responsibilities of your own life and those of caregiving, and are team-oriented, then you may be a sharing caregiver. Having another family member or two available to handle what needs to get done increases balance and is more advantageous for all parties involved. It's always easier to carry a heavy load with assistance. This works best if the family members live relatively close to each other and to the parent.

My younger sister and I live in separate cities, three hours apart. Travelling, when required, was not impossible, but it could become inconvenient. You cannot reasonably expect a sibling to drive several hours into town just to transport your parent to the doctor, pick up required medications, help tend to other needs, and allow you respite time. Mind you, if one sibling is being asked repeatedly to run the necessary errands simply because he or she is the closest, then this individual should be compensated in some manner (e.g., a regular gas fill-up for his or her vehicle would be appreciated). Your parent may require more immediate treatment that cannot wait. As this caregiving arrangement requires working together and compromising, siblings should also be on friendly terms.

3.3 Collaborative caregiver

A collaborative caregiver is practical, sensible, realistic, and resourceful. Consider yourself very lucky if you fall into this category. Similar to a sharing caregiver, a collaborative caregiver will participate as a caregiver; however, he or she will have the necessary resources to call on many others to work together to provide proper care. Many of these individuals and outside services can be identified by using the Your Circle of Caregiving worksheet, located at the end of this book. For example, collaborative caregivers may rely on the nursing staff at a long-term care facility, a private companion, an activity coordinator who plans specialized outings for seniors, or a respite group that takes the parent for the day.

As the old saying goes, "Many hands make light work." As a collaborative caregiver, you will find you can better handle what is required and benefit from some regular time away yourself. If you are not a collaborative caregiver, work toward becoming one. Doing so is certainly advantageous because it will benefit both your own physical and mental health. You will not be as busy or emotionally taxed. Such an arrangement helps you to reduce your own stress and workload.

3.4 Coordinating caregiver

Are you the type of person that researches, analyzes, and organizes everything? That would mean you fall into the category of the coordinating caregiver. You will spend much of your time learning about relevant matters and then deciding on the best course of action. You will collect data and compare options such as researching medical advances, learning the possible side effects of prescribed medications, visiting long-term care facilities and assessing their suitability, or evaluating different models of motorized scooters.

I tend to scribble things down on spare pieces of paper and then promptly lose them, so I would not make an effective coordinating caregiver; to be a coordinating caregiver, you must be highly organized. You will have (perhaps colour-coded) files for everything, you will keep brochures together, and you will remember to take receipts out of your shirt pockets before laundering!

3.5 Delegating caregiver

The delegating caregiver is the type of person who is dynamic, confident, and a leader. This individual is the least hands-on because he or she assigns and hires others to provide the necessary care. You may be uncomfortable with the necessary tasks or realize that others are infinitely more qualified to do this than you are.

I see myself as a delegate as my professional background does not include anything resembling health care. I shied away from certain tasks (e.g., I balked at the very idea of giving either of my parents a bath). Assigning certain responsibilities to me would have been both inappropriate and unsafe for my parents. Delegating caregivers often are more financially able to hire the extra help.

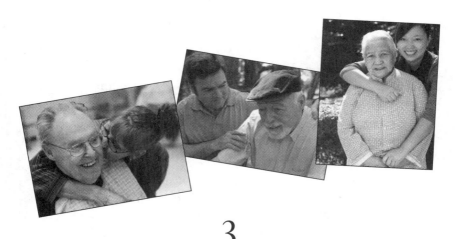

3

CAREGIVING FROM A DISTANCE

"You give but little when you give of your possessions.
It is when you give of yourself that you truly give."

KAHLIL GIBRAN

Families often drift apart geographically, which can make caregiving more difficult. An outstretched hand can only reach so far. While caregiving from afar is possible, it becomes more expensive and distant family caregivers do pay the price. In the news article, "Caring for elderly parents from afar takes toll on time, money: StatsCan," a research study involving 23,000 Canadian respondents aged 45 or older, found that "about 62 percent of long-distance caregivers taking care of elderly parents incurred extra expenses, compared to 30 percent of those who live nearby."

For the purposes of the StatsCan study, a "long-distance caregiver" is one who lives further than one hour's drive from his or her aging parents. Realize that one hour is doubled to account for the return trip home and two hours on the road is almost 10 percent of a day. This report continues by explaining that travelling time and financial costs both increase dramatically. Those surveyed that lived more than half a day away from their elderly parents were much more likely to miss full days of work than those surveyed that lived in the same neighbourhood as their parents. The survey also noted that the people that lived far away from their parents spent three times the amount of money on caregiving than those who lived close to their parents.

Family caregivers can be caught between a rock and a hard place. Should they be expected to pay out-of-pocket for expenses incurred? No. Will family caregivers continue to cover these costs? Until family caregivers can be subsidized somehow for the work they do, they will be responsible for the costs.

Warmer temperatures, like those on Canada's west coast, have great appeal for older people, but rural life can also be attractive to seniors. Smaller towns offer a more relaxed way of life and a closer-knit community feel; yet, they can fall short when it comes to necessary care and resources. The nearest doctor may be an hour's drive away. The local hospital may not be prepared for all medical emergencies.

In my case, my parents retired from their previous, often chilly, family home where they had lived for 25 years to the much warmer Victoria, British Columbia. I can't say that I blamed them for wanting to move there; however, my sisters and I quickly realized that Mom and Dad did not have much personal or professional support on Vancouver Island. This became painfully obvious when Mom needed immediate medical care. With her low hemoglobin counts, Mom was urged by her physician to check into the hospital. Reportedly, she struggled physically to reach the hospital — stumbling down the street and often clasping on to street lamps for support.

We didn't know anything about this until my younger sister got a phone call from a social worker from the hospital. Mom, bless her soul, was concerned about leaving Dad alone at home. My younger sister, being the most available, immediately booked a flight and arrived shortly to tend to Mom and Dad's needs. Fortunately, her schedule allowed her some flexibility and she was able to do this without much difficulty. You may not be as lucky. Your employer may be resistant about giving you time off on short notice or you may have your own family obligations.

1. THE CHALLENGES OF LONG-DISTANCE CAREGIVING

I found that long-distance caregiving comes with many challenges. Most prevalent are the financial costs (e.g., long-distance telephone bills and travelling expenses), which can skyrocket for distant family members. Frequently, caregivers pay for these expenses out of their own pockets — doing so can regrettably lead to resentment toward parents, the situation, and other siblings who may be blamed for not fully carrying their weight. Finding the best ways to save money and time may help reduce the resentment.

1.1 Communication

Even from a distance, communication is possible. The telephone and postal services are old familiar standbys, but also consider the Internet. If your parents are tech-savvy, you can set up a webcam. With this, you may speak to and see your loved ones in real time. An email can be composed, sent, and received within mere minutes. Relevant website links, detailing important health information or otherwise, can be shared. You can easily forward digital family photos. These can be snapped, transformed into computer files, and sent electronically. Digitized information can be sent from you to your parents but also between your other siblings. A weekly email report summarizing your parent's latest news can be sent to siblings who live elsewhere. Such news can be comforting and often enough to keep other family members involved.

Something you may want to consider is Skype, which is a computer program where you can call, video call, and instant message each other for free. Note that as with anything new, your loved one must be comfortable using technology. Unfortunately, many seniors resist learning about computers due to uncertainty, rigidity, or fear. Know and respect your parents' limits. Keep in mind, too, your parents' limiting factors — although my dad had relied on a computer for his work, eventually he completely forgot how to operate one.

When considering long-distance phone calls, limiting your calls to off-peak hours may seem easy enough; however, this cannot realistically happen. Many of the businesses, service centres, and doctors' offices that you will need to contact may not be open past 6:00 p.m. or on the weekend. With caregiving, you can never guarantee that your phone calls will only be required on evenings and weekends or at your own convenience. You may be operating around the clock; however, business owners do not always recognize this same need.

A mobile phone does, despite additional airtime charges, have a distinct advantage for a caregiver. I am speaking of the added convenience; you can place a call or be called almost anywhere. When I used my cell phone for such purposes, I referred to it as my "caregiving hotline" as I could be immediately reached.

With my mobile phone, I was offered the often-standard "free evenings and weekends" feature. I could make local calls between 5:00 p.m. and 6:00 a.m., Monday to Friday as well as all day on Saturday and Sunday, at no additional charge. Of the numerous airtime packages available, I then chose a basic deal for cost-savings. If you use more minutes than what is agreed on in the sales contract, you will pay a cost per minute or second. Be careful of this clause as you may be overcharged — should you talk for one minute and 15 seconds extra, you could be charged for two minutes.

If you are shopping for a cell phone to carry with you, I recommend that you shop around for the best deals. With the plans varying dramatically, consider them all carefully and ask yourself what works best for you. Think about your own phone usage — will you really need 500-plus free daytime minutes monthly?

My cell phone included a few additional features, which I found handy when serving as a caregiver. Consider the following options. With voicemail, callers can leave a message. Just as with a regular landline phone, you may not always be available to answer the call. Call display shows the incoming caller's name and phone number. If I was busy with Mom or Dad at the time a call came through, I could quickly glance at my phone and decide whether or not to answer or let it ring through to voicemail. Call forwarding transfers incoming calls from one number to another. This feature I found repeatedly useful as people could still reach me when I was away from home. Know that these little "extras" do cost extra; however, they can be well worth it. Another practical tool is a car-charging cord for your cell phone; with this you may recharge a dwindling phone battery even when you are away from home.

Don't ever get persuaded into buying more accessories than you find absolutely necessary. A popular sales gimmick is to offer the cell phone at very little or no charge and then lock the customer into a long-term airtime contract. Such contracts can be difficult to break, unless you are willing to buy out the remaining time on your term. Carefully evaluate the length of the contract term. Will a longer term remain appropriate for your needs? Instead, look into "pay as you go" plans to avoid such an obligation; here, a customer will deposit money into a plan and withdraw on this to make calls. Doing this is an ideal way to keep a better handle on your spending. On the downside, you may overlook depositing into your account and temporarily lose service, just when you may need it the most.

If you are shopping for a new or replacement cell phone, do confirm that you will have service coverage where you will be, or plan to be, physically located — if there aren't any transmission towers in your area, a cell phone is of no use. Service is generally quite good in urban areas, and it's always improving across the nation — but while driving to the west coast on caregiving business, I was unreachable through sections of the Rocky Mountains. Make sure you will be in a strong service area the majority of the time before purchasing a cell phone.

Another issue to look into is "roaming charges" where you can be charged extra for long-distance calls made both to and from your mobile telephone, when you are outside of your coverage area.

You may also wish to consider not sharing this phone number with your entire social circle. This way you won't have the line tied up with unnecessary calls; instead, you know the incoming calls will most likely be caregiving-related.

Keep your conversations on your mobile phone short. While you may be tempted to chat at greater detail about matters-at-hand, remember that you are paying for the convenience of the service. The extra minutes can add up quickly. Mobile phones are also not always best for private conversations; for example, if you have ever ridden in an elevator or sat beside someone on the bus who is talking on his or her phone about personal issues, you know how uncomfortable and distracting this can be. Therefore, if you take a call pertaining to confidential matters, there is nothing wrong with asking your caller to hold a few moments until you find a quiet corner to talk. Alternatively, you can explain that you cannot talk right now but you will phone back. Be polite but firm with callers; just because they have reached you on your cellular telephone, it does not mean that you are necessarily able to chat freely.

Keep your home landline phone, by all means, but investigate long-distance calling plans with your own telephone company. My older sister was lucky to find a package offering unlimited calling for one monthly flat rate, and we made very good use of this. Don't wait for your telephone company to advertise a calling bundle. Instead, call the company and inquire about cost-saving measures.

You may also want to consider booking a conference call involving a handful of people in a caregiving conversation. Instructions for conference calling can often be found in the first few pages of your local telephone directory. An advantage here is that all persons involved do not have to be in the same room. If this is impossible, gather your caregivers together in a home with numerous phone jacks. My older sister has three telephones in her home; this arrangement worked well for the family. If these are cordless telephones, you can sit closer to each other and converse more effectively.

An alternative to conference calls is to use a speakerphone. You can collect your local circle of caregivers in one room and still involve someone far away. To remain effective, participants should be encouraged to take turns speaking. We've all been in busy rooms with several conversations going on simultaneously; it is very easy to lose track of what is being said.

By using a speakerphone, several people chiming in on a conversation can easily create chaos. Emotions can run high during such conversations and participants may forget and just "jump in" to the conversation. Should you be recording these conversations, you'll also want to recommend to everybody present to be very cognizant of not speaking when someone else is. You may want to appoint a moderator to help maintain control. You could also ask everyone in the room you're in to raise their hands when they wish to say something. For the best sound quality when recording, try to choose a distraction-free room that has a low ceiling. Close the door to reduce outside noise or any pets or children wandering in at inopportune moments.

If someone cannot attend, you could also record these conversations and send the person a copy of the recording. By using a digital tape recorder, sessions can be recorded, uploaded to a computer, and emailed as an audio file.

To take this idea a step further, you could even record caregiving updates (involving more general, less time-sensitive information) and send these electronically to other family members who couldn't attend the meeting. Obviously, doing this will save on long-distance phone bills; the recipient will receive these immediately and can also listen at his or her convenience and replay the recording to clarify any missed information. You may want to keep these recordings for future use; for example, maybe your family wants to capture your parent's story for future generations, or in the unfortunate event of a conflict, a record can prove immeasurably useful.

1.2 Frequent travel

Frequent travelling to visit a loved one can prove to be costly. Unlike booking a flight for a holiday, depending on your parent's situation, you won't necessarily have the luxury of pre-shopping months in advance for the least expensive airfare. Much like my younger sister did, you may well have to travel at a moment's notice when emergency strikes. With flying, costs typically rise closer to the weekend and nearing holidays (e.g., Christmas). Even the price of gas typically increases just before a long weekend.

One creative way to save money on flights is to cash in your collected "frequent flyer" miles, which are offered as incentives with different credit cards. The cardholder is awarded points, proportionate to purchases, which can be cashed in on air travel costs. Such frequent flyer points can add up quickly. These points can often be redeemed quite simply and may be transferable (therefore, you may be able to "gift" your points to another family member to use instead).

Furthermore, travelling to a distant city or town will take time away from your own family and/or work (which can affect your income). For my sisters and I, flying to Victoria took a couple of hours. Ask yourself if you will always have that kind of time available.

Boarding a bus or riding a train are other viable means of transportation. While you will be more restricted by a carrier's schedule, you can still travel between points and save on your own vehicle expenses.

If you live closer to your parents, you can always drive; however, you will need to consider the fuel costs and the wear-and-tear on your vehicle, not to mention the personal wear-and-tear on you. Driving long distances can be quite physically and mentally taxing. Should you be driving extensive distances on lonely highways, remember to top up your gas tank before leaving home and keep your fully charged cellular phone in your glove compartment in case of emergencies.

No matter where you live in this country, Canadian winters can be harsh. If you are driving, pack a few extra layers of clothing, a shovel, a blanket or sleeping bag, candles, and matches. No matter what time of year you are driving, don't forget to also take some extra provisions to eat and drink.

Check the spare tire for proper inflation and understand how to use your car's jack. With longer-distance driving, ensure that your car is regularly serviced and leave a planned itinerary with someone back home. If you are unfamiliar with the route, map it before you go or use a GPS system to direct you.

If you travel to visit your parent, you will be busy. This isn't a vacation. If you do not have your own vehicle, rent one when you arrive. Weigh the alternatives carefully; for example, if you have a great deal of running around to do, a compact car will be less expensive on gas costs; however, a larger car will be more comfortable for your parent if he or she is riding with you. Consider the practicality of the vehicle. A four-door model will be more spacious, a larger trunk can better hold a folded wheelchair, and a fold-down back seat in a hatchback can provide additional luggage space.

You may also want to incorporate some fun into your rental vehicle. On one trip to Victoria, I rented a vintage Volkswagen Beetle. Mom, having driven one of these herself in the past, was quite tickled to be shuttled around in the "bug" and to relive her memories.

If possible, sign for a rental plan where you will not be charged per kilometer. Note that the extra insurance costs for a rental vehicle may not be necessary. Check with your own insurance agent back home to see if your coverage will also include a second car. If you have a major credit card, additional insurance may be available; this can be well worth looking into.

Given the options, driving your own car may be the preferred choice. The benefits here are that your own car will be most familiar to you as the driver and you will be guaranteed to have a vehicle to use at your destination. There will be no hassles trying to find a car to rent when you get there, or having to accept another make or model of vehicle because your preferred method is unavailable.

1.3 Travelling with your parent

Should you and your parent travel together, inquire about a companion fare. Frequently, transportation carriers offer a discounted rate on a second seat to someone accompanying a senior. If you are successful in negotiating a less expensive fare, know that other senior-friendly services may also be offered. Airlines will often allow those passengers "requiring assistance" to board the airplane first.

Airlines may also loan you a narrowed wheelchair, which allows for better maneuverability inside the airplane.

You can also combine your transportation to ease travel stress. I remember a family trip to Mount Rainier, one of my mother's most-admired mountain peaks. My two sisters, along with my niece and nephew, drove the entire distance while I flew halfway with Mom and Dad and then rented a car to drive the remaining distance. What sounded like making a trip more complicated than necessary worked out well. We knew that both Mom and Dad would not be comfortable making the long road trip, especially with two raucous kids in the car, so the combination of flying and driving worked for our situation. We also had the luxury of having two vehicles, rather than one, at our destination. As the trip required extensive walking and Mom couldn't be on her feet a great deal, we rented a wheelchair from our local Red Cross office. This proved to be the ideal answer.

Before you and your loved one fly together, confirm with a doctor that it safe to do so. High altitudes can make breathing difficult. Your parent must be medically cleared. Will medications need to be taken during the flight? If so, can you bring said medications onboard with you? What about additional health-care apparatus? An oxygen tank, for example, may be available in a reduced size for ease of transport. If you are unsure on these matters, don't just assume that everything will be fine. Call ahead to your airline or discuss it with your travel agent and confirm what the exact rules are for flying. What medications and medical apparatuses can be brought onboard? Should you have to fly repeatedly for caregiving business, double-check with the airline that these same rules apply with each trip you take.

Another thing to consider is whether your parent can last the entire flight without going to the bathroom. Ushering an unsteady senior from his or her seat to the rear of the plane to squeeze into closet-sized facilities is certainly anything but ideal. You should consider whether movement will be required; if so, seat your loved one next to the aisle rather than by the window. As with medications and medical apparatuses, you can talk to the airline company or the travel agent. Instead of reserving an aisle seat somewhere in the middle of the plane (a tactic I will often employ to guarantee the most legroom possible), perhaps it is possible to book a seat closer to the washroom to alleviate any of your parent's discomfort?

While little can be done to improve a passenger's comfort in tighter quarters, you can pack along a neck pillow and an extra blanket. Even a tightly rolled towel or jacket, tucked in between a person's back and the seat, can provide necessary stability and cushioning. Both you and your loved one will be more comfortable for travelling if you dress in looser fitting clothes. You may even want to tuck an extra change of clothes into a carry-on bag for your parent. For longer flights where a meal may be served, confirm ahead of time that any dietary restrictions will be addressed.

Another prerequisite for travelling with seniors is a checklist. Without wanting to sound harsh, don't rely on aging memories to try and remember details. Draft up a list and check it yourself to confirm everything is taken care of. Double-check the contents of your parent's suitcase, or better yet, pack it yourself to ensure that nothing is left behind.

At times like these, you cannot always trust your own memory either. With caregiving, you will often have a great deal of facts to remember. Due to these stressful circumstances, you may not remember flight times, airline numbers, or your own suitcase. A checklist can also help you to stay organized and help reduce your stress.

In addition to packing your suitcases for the trip, remember to pack along plenty of patience. With slower-moving seniors, you must allow for ample time to leave home, at stopover points, and at your final destination. Confirm prior to arriving at transfer points that you will have enough time. Are your arrival and departure gates at the airport on completely opposite sides of the terminal? Can assistance be offered for seniors to reduce the need to walk? You may be able to borrow a wheelchair. Some airports I have been in use golf carts to shuttle passengers and luggage. If you are driving, you may want to map out regular rest stops to get out of the car, walk around, stretch, and go to the bathroom.

1.4 Finding accommodations

Guest accommodation for visiting caregivers must also be addressed. Where will you stay when you arrive? Many newer seniors' apartment buildings now feature guest suites, which is a clever idea where visiting family members can stay on a temporary basis. Considering the alternative of booking a few nights in a local hotel, this option is far more cost-effective, comfortable, and convenient.

A visiting caregiver can also scope out the building and witness the staff at work. This can provide you more peace-of-mind. If space permits, you can always "camp out" with your parents. My mother and father's home in Victoria fortunately had a spare room. Without an extra bed or even a couch though, a visiting sibling would be relegated to a sleeping bag with a couch pillow on the floor. For the convenience and comfort of visiting family caregivers, you could store an inflatable mattress, an extra pillow, and a few blankets in a closet.

If you do prefer a real bed, locate a hotel or motel nearby. As with airline flights, know that your credit card's frequent flyer points will often cover a percentage of your accommodation costs. The Canadian Automobile Association (CAA) offers a similar incentive to its members. If you are working with a travel agent, inquire about package deals in which you can book a flight, a hotel room, and a rental car for a better deal. Shop around. Can the price of travel be reduced if you stay over a weekend? While these reward points typically cannot be used over holidays (airlines prefer to save plane seats for paying passengers), there are ample opportunities to take advantage of this offer throughout the rest of the year.

Should you expect to be visiting your parent often and staying in the same hotel repeatedly, get to know the hotel manager and explain that you will be a regular guest. As such, you may well be able to negotiate a better price for a few nights' stay or perhaps an upgrade to a larger room. It never hurts to ask about an offered discount either. Many times hotels will offer you a better rate if they are not booked solid. For the hotel manager, getting even partial payment for a room is better than having that room sit empty.

2. WHAT TO DO WHEN YOU GET THERE

After arriving, ensure that you meet your parent's neighbours and friends. Exchange phone numbers with them, because these individuals can provide a much-needed set of helpful eyes and ears after you are gone. Also consider providing your parent's trusted neighbours with an extra set of keys to use in case of any urgent situation.

Attend as many area functions with your parent as possible during your visit. This will get your parent out and active within the local community. Help your parent join a seniors' centre, which can offer friendships and activities. Suggest classes or workshops that your parent may be interested in taking; instructors may be willing to welcome your parent in to simply audit a class for no credit. Investigate local volunteering opportunities where your parent could share his or her experience with others.

When my mother and father lived in Victoria, they got involved with Meals on Wheels. This is a program that prepares and provides meals to housebound seniors. My parents volunteered as drivers which worked out very well for many reasons — doing this involved them in the community, it kept them both active, it allowed them to meet others, and it provided a chance to better learn their way around their new city. Mom and Dad would have appreciated the opportunity to give back and would have felt valued.

If your parent has religious beliefs, attend church services with him or her. You could ask among the congregation if home visits can be arranged, or, if someone from the church can call every few days to check in on your parent.

Look into local service providers such as a regular housekeeper to come in to clean, launder clothes, and perform other light household duties. This can be of immense help, not to mention the person can provide some welcome company for your parents. That same housekeeper may also be called on to cook meals if that is a service he or she provides.

You may also want to consider hiring someone or finding a volunteer that will mow your parent's lawn or shovel snow. Not only does this reduce the heavier work for your mother or father, it also reduces the risk of injuries incurred. For example, your parent may easily slip and fall on a snow-covered sidewalk while trying to clear away ice and snow.

Securing a home-care service to provide regular help with dressing or bathing your parent may also be something you need to consider. More seniors' services are being offered on a mobile basis; professionals can come to your parent's home to provide haircutting, glasses repair, dentistry, or pedicures. Check your local phone book, make some calls, and inquire into the availability of such services.

2.1 Find the necessary information and documents

Meet all the professionals currently involved with your parent's care. The professionals may include a doctor, lawyer, and banker. During my visits to see my parents, I always packed along a notebook and a couple of pens — having more than one pen meant I would always have an extra, should the other run out of ink at an inopportune moment. When I met with the banker, investment advisor, doctor, and realtor, I always made copious notes of our conversations. In addition, I found the notebook handy to record thoughts, observances (e.g., maybe Mom was more tired today than yesterday or Dad had remembered what day of the week it was), and questions I should ask. When it comes to asking questions, keep doing so until you completely understand the answers. You are doing this on your loved one's behalf: Advocate and clarify. Don't be embarassed if you don't completely understand; professionals of all types often speak in industry jargon which, unless you have gained related knowledge, you often cannot comprehend.

When talking to the banker, collect necessary banking information such as the bank location, account number, and value of additional investment holdings. Don't overlook any foreign accounts and credit cards!

Confirm the whereabouts of all necessary documents such as the will, birth certificate, Social Insurance cards, and health-care cards and ensure these are kept secure. A common holding spot for these documents is a bank safety deposit box, so make sure you ask for an extra key to take back home with you. If there is no bank safety deposit box, purchase a small, fireproof safe for home storage. As an extra precaution, photocopy all the documents you find and keep these copies at a separate, safe location; you never know when you might need them.

The Caregiver's Document Worksheet found at the end of this book will help you gather all the information you need.

2.2 Check the safety of your parent's home

When you are visiting, also remain alert to the safety issues of your parent's home — both the interior and the exterior. Frayed or loose carpeting can be a dangerous tripping hazard. Extra furniture may only occupy space and not serve any useful purpose.

Observe your parent getting in and out of his or her chair; if extensive effort is required, maybe it is time to replace this furniture? While it can be difficult to dismiss any sentimental attachments you may have to an old couch or rocking chair, do so. If you, or another family member, choose not to adopt your parent's furniture, it is far better to sell, donate, or even discard tables, chairs, and shelves rather than place them in storage indefinitely. The monthly fee for secured lock-up can add up quickly. Save yourself the money and call on local nonprofit associations, they may be able to find a good home for your parent's old armchair. Better yet, maybe they will even arrange pick-up.

Check for any lightbulbs that need to be replaced. You may find that you need to install a new lighting fixture to remove dangerous shadows in the hallway — aging eyes aren't quite as sharp as they once were. You may need to remove a mirror at the end of the hall — even a somewhat cognitively impaired senior may be startled or confused to see another person walking toward him or her.

Check for leaks in the roof or around windows or doors. Replace broken windows, which can allow for cold air to enter the home. Walk around your parent's home; verify that the smoke alarm is working properly.

Pay close attention to the bathroom — with wet floors, this can become a deathtrap. Install grab bars around the shower and bathtub. Place a non-skid mat in the shower and tub. Replace flooring, if necessary, and avoid slippery tiles. Invest in a walk-in bathtub where the senior can step in, sit down, close the door, and enjoy a good soak. A jacuzzi bathtub's hot water jets can be very therapeutic for sore joints and nagging injuries.

Are there stairs inside or outside the home? Explore the possibility of installing a mechanical stair-lift, which can smoothly carry your loved one up or down a flight of stairs. Without access to a basement or second level of a home, that area becomes wasted space. Alternatively, consider if a wheelchair ramp can be placed at the front, side, or rear of the home. If land space is limited, a wheelchair ramp does not have to extend straight out; it can be built to double back on itself or even curl around. Just ensure that the incline is not too steep and that the ramp features secure handrails, so that your parents can pull themselves up, if need be.

Homes should not only be comfortable for the resident, they must also be safe. Be fully prepared to make any adaptations necessary for your parent's safety. While you may hesitate to pay a lot for home reconstruction, do know that many of these necessary changes will increase your property's value. Look for a qualified contractor to complete any extensive modifications, check references, and get written estimates prior to the work being started.

At the end of this book, you will find the Home Safety Checklist to help you make sure your loved one is safe and has ease of mobility in his or her own home.

3. RESPECT THE DECISION THAT NOT EVERYONE WANTS TO RELOCATE

I was lucky that when my parents' medical situations arose, my mother and father understood the need to return to Alberta even though it was not their dream retirement destination. They realized and accepted that the move was for the best.

Should your parents remain obstinate, please take a page out of my family's caregiving manual and share the workload with your other relatives, if possible. In my case, my sisters and I rotated as a full-time caregiver for Mom and Dad in Victoria, prior to their move back to Alberta. This idea, resulting in each of us taking a temporary leave from work to focus on our parents' needs, evolved from ongoing discussion. Prior to receiving the scheduled evening phone calls, I would take a few minutes and review my notes from the day. We made very good use of my older sister's flat-rate long-distance calling plan during that time!

Your parents may not be as obliging as mine were. If your mother and father do not wish to move, there is little you can do about it. In this case, the need for long-distance caregiving practices and open lines of communication become even more necessary. Hiring a part-time or full-time local caregiver to help is a viable option. A job requirement for a distant caregiver could be to participate in a weekly conference call to you and your siblings to share any news or concerns, which may help to provide you with peace of mind.

In addition to being your eyes and ears from afar, hired caregivers can also work in another important role. When you visit your parent, you can ask your hired help to run some necessary errands, thus freeing up your time so you may relax more with your parent.

If, however, your parent's (or your own) finances are limited, you may not be able to afford private care. In this case, can you relocate yourself, even temporarily, to help tend to parental needs? Openly discuss your need for a leave of absence with your employer. You may be able to negotiate a discount with a local hotel if you wish to stay long-term; however, you may be far more comfortable renting an apartment for three to six months, or more if necessary. For furnishings, you can rent furniture — items can be delivered, and picked up when you no longer require them. You may also have the option of renting a furnished apartment.

Aging parents are not the only ones who move away. Adult children can relocate as well. This may be done for any number of reasons such as a job offer, a blossoming relationship, educational training, or simply due to personal preference. Respect a person's choice to move away. While you can reasonably request a person's involvement with caregiving responsibilities, you must also respect his or her choice to remain distant.

Someone may resist becoming more involved due to personal discomfort with a situation. While I was okay with handling Mom and Dad's banking, I hesitated to give either of them a bath. Not only was this uncomfortable for me, it would have posed great danger for my parents. Without the necessary medical experience, I have never been trained in proper individual lifting and transferring techniques. It is far better to delegate such tasks to a qualified health-care worker. Involve someone in caregiving only as much as this individual chooses to help and is able to do so.

4. EMOTIONAL DISTANCE

In addition to physical distance, caregivers can experience emotional distance. For any number of personal reasons, family members may feel uncomfortable stepping into a caregiver's shoes. In such cases, do not force anyone to take on a job unwillingly. A reluctant caregiver is a resistant caregiver and one not helpful to your situation. Caregiving requires ability, desire, trust, and dedication, so if a sibling does not want to help out, it's best to accept this and carry on.

Arguing is often pointless and can only drive a dagger deeper into teetering family relationships. Instead, talk openly with the other person, understand his or her reasons for the decision, and be accepting. Often, these reasons will be quite sound. It remains best to involve someone in your family only as much as he or she wants to become involved. Try compromising to avoid family hostility. It's better to accept the familial differences now than to face possible alienation later.

When working closely with other family members, expect to encounter opposition. You are all at very close quarters at these times and not everybody may agree that one approach is the best direction to take. Consensus may be more difficult to reach than you might imagine. There were a number of heated discussions that occurred between my sisters and I; however, we eventually decided to accept other points of view, negotiate, and compromise.

Arguing might well occur within your own family, but you must remember that caregiving is not all about you: It is about your loved one. Know that you do not have to win all the arguments, suggest the best option, or be right every time. Park your own pride and ask yourself the following questions:

- How will your parent best benefit?
- What is important to your parent?
- What values does he or she hold dear?
- What would he or she do in a similar situation?

Considering what your parent would do in a similar situation helps to put you in his or her perspective. In making the same choice your parent would, it will help to put your parent more at ease. With caregiving, you don't want your parent or siblings to feel threatened or become defensive. This will make caregiving even more challenging. Thinking in parental terms may make difficult family decisions easier, and can often be more beneficial in the long term.

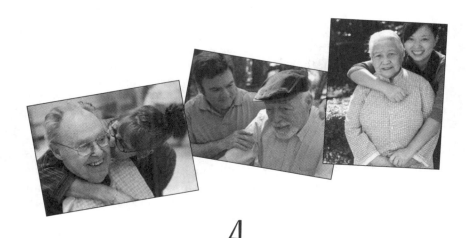

4
FINDING AND MOVING YOUR PARENT INTO SUITABLE ACCOMMODATIONS

"Home is a shelter from storms — all sorts of storms."
WILLIAM J. BENNETT

The move is imminent. Your parent has weakened, become sick, or has outgrown offered services in some other way. Where your parent will go depends on his or her current and future needs. Different levels of care exist so you must ensure that you make the proper choice — the facility must be suitable for the immediate situation.

Know that this time can be immensely trying for caregivers. When I helped to move my father into long-term care, the stark reality hit me hard that he was not going to get better — it had to be done.

1. THE DIFFERENT TYPES OF LIVING ARRANGEMENTS

No matter where you live in Canada and whether you are new to caregiving or well-established in this role, you will hear various terms for seniors' living choices. Where does one begin?

Essentially, there are three key steps to choosing the right place and finding comfort that you have chosen well:

1. **Evaluate your parent's needs, wants, and resources.** By carefully considering your parent's current physical and mental capabilities, as well as what may potentially lie ahead, you are

45

well on your way to selecting an appropriate setting for your mother or father. Ask your parent's doctor for a complete medical diagnosis and appropriate accommodation recommendations so you can be prepared. If your parent remains cognitively aware, ask him or her about living preferences and then seek out living options.

Ask yourself: Will your parent be happy living at this facility? Know that your parent may balk at even hearing the idea of moving into long-term care, but he or she may become much happier and healthier as a result of admission. Understand that there are costs involved with continuing care facilities (of any kind); can your parent or the family incur these costs without financial hardship? Are there any hidden costs (e.g., to cover a private room or additional care)? Look at your parent's entire financial picture (e.g., accumulated savings in his or her bank account, investments, building and property holdings, and continued income such as through a pension). How likely are these costs to rise over the next few years and by how much? Can your family or your parent afford all types of care in the long term?

2. **Evaluate your options.** By visiting each facility you are considering (by all means, take your parent along and ask for his or her opinion), you can collect a great deal of information. Compare your findings carefully. Is the level of care appropriate? Does your parent like the facility? Where is the property located? What amenities are offered? What is the cost of care? Negotiation on a final choice may be called for amongst you and your family. Know that this negotiation can only be done when your parent remains well and more independent. Fewer choices exist as your parent ages and declines. Once I was faced with moving Dad into a secured Alzheimer's unit, there was little I could do — my sisters and I were resigned to accepting the first bed that became available for him.

3. **Shortlist your top choices.** This process can be very similar to a job interview where you will personally meet with the most likely candidates, perhaps call them back for a second interview, and then hire the best candidate. The key here is the personal contact. You can learn much more about a person during a face-to-face meeting than you can by speaking to him or her on the telephone. What this means to you is that you must personally visit each potential facility option so

as to make the best, the most logical, and the most educated decision for your mother or father.

With diverse care options available — including independent living, assisted living, continuing care, and many more — it is easy enough for caregivers to be confused as to where to place their aging mother or father to receive the best care. To make matters even more complicated, there can be a great deal of crossover in services provided between care facilities.

How do you know which facility will provide the best care possible for your parent? How much care will be required in the future? This question in particular is a difficult one to answer because nothing is certain. But, by thoroughly researching the specific health condition, you can have a better idea of what can be expected. Trying to define and differentiate between all the lifestyle options available can be enough to make your head spin. Therefore, I will focus on several of the key terms you will likely hear as your parent's condition progresses. For further clarification, I have ranked these in your parent's likely order of need.

1.1 Home care

Home care consists of support services that can be provided to seniors who remain living in their own homes. The types of support services can vary dramatically, depending on a senior's needs. Your mother could be bathed and clothed in the mornings; your father could be shaved and have his lunch prepared for him. Home-care workers can provide an increased level of comfort for distant family caregivers who will know that someone is stopping by to check on their parent to ensure everything is okay.

When it comes to having your parent assessed by a home-care association, know that your vision of what is needed may differ dramatically from what is actually offered. For example, while perhaps you believe that your parent requires five baths per week, your parent may only be bathed three times per week. Also note your parent may not have the same home-care worker visit each time, which may cause undue confusion or anxiety.

1.2 Independent living

As the term "independent living" implies, these types of facilities are ideal for seniors who can still live and function quite well on their own. Your mother or father will typically live in an apartment-style place (i.e., either a studio or a one-bedroom unit) with kitchen facilities and a small fridge. Residents can typically choose between renting or buying a unit and home-care services can be provided.

1.3 Supportive living

When your parent begins to lose physical or cognitive abilities, he or she should be transferred to more of a supportive lifestyle environment. Much like independent living, these properties consist of individual apartments but also feature various common areas, shared by the residents (e.g., a library, a recreation room, or a craft room). The primary difference here is that supportive-living facilities offer enhanced security to the resident and the resident's family through around-the-clock emergency response, as well as the convenience of prepared meals and housekeeping services. A full-time doctor or registered nurse is usually not required; staff will consist of personal-care aides who provide limited support.

1.4 Assisted living

There are similarities and crossover in services offered between supportive and assisted living for seniors. With assisted living, a senior can receive more hands-on health care and management. Staff in assisted-living facilities can assist with medication reminders and delivery, and bathing and dressing a resident. Such personal care can become uncomfortable, tricky, and risky for family caregivers to provide; therefore, you can expect to find more qualified health-care professionals onsite. As an example, a licensed practical nurse will have the experience and know-how to be able to competently dispense medications, give shots, and take temperatures, while a personal-care aide can only serve in lesser duties (e.g., accompanying your parent on a walk or feeding him or her).

1.5 Long-term care

A long-term care facility is often the final stop for a senior who has advanced-health issues. Long-term care facilities are staffed full-time by practiced health-care professionals who competently provide any number of required care services to a senior. Rooms in this type of facility are either private or shared and there is little privacy for residents. With such facilities, the senior or family caregiver will pay a monthly fee to cover the cost of care.

Obviously, at this advanced level of care, home-care services are not required. At my father's long-term care facility, one Registered

Nurse was always on duty to implement resident care plans and oversee operations.

2. THINGS TO CONSIDER WHEN SEARCHING FOR ACCOMMODATIONS FOR YOUR PARENT

Finding the right accommodations for your parent may cause some confusion because there remains a great deal of crossover between each type of care facility. Similar to my situation, you may be required to move your parent one or more times. Moving a senior can often be very challenging; you might doubt that you are making the best decision, and you might face resistance from your parent who may fear what lies ahead.

Looking at long-term care options is daunting for caregivers. I almost envied my father, who was not even aware of the forthcoming moves and the amount of work involved. As a caregiver, you should not jump into a decision too hastily because with poor judgment, both you and your parent can be negatively affected. You've likely heard the expression, "when you fail to plan, you plan to fail." This is true. By failing to plan properly, your parent could be receiving inadequate care, paying excessive care costs, or living in a less-than-ideal facility.

My best advice is to tour the facilities of choice and ask pointed questions. When I was inquiring about the available facilities for my dad, I discovered that a lot of the properties only offered group tours which were scheduled once or twice per week. If at all possible, you should push for an independent tour. While group tours may be more convenient for care-centre staff, the times and dates may not be convenient for you and you do not have to be totally obliging. In addition, with being part of a group tour, you may get hustled through the property before you have a chance to ask all of your questions. Although you may feel uncomfortable raising certain questions, you have every right to ask questions and find out the answers before you make a decision.

Don't just settle for the mapped-out tour where you will only see what is shown. Investigate less-populated areas including stairwells and closets; are these swept and mopped regularly? Ask to see the kitchen and food-service areas. Is this a healthy and sanitary environment? Are the public washrooms cleaned?

Don't overlook how accommodating the facility will be to your parent's lifestyle. What I mean by this is, does your parent have any idiosyncrasies that may require addressing? As an example, both my mother and father enjoyed sipping a glass of wine with their dinner — a harmless enough matter — yet, we had to pass on several independent living properties with communal resident dining where management was not comfortable with any alcohol consumption at all.

To better prepare yourself for the choice ahead, you will want to speak with other family members of the residents. As a casual visitor, you will face resistance from the staff if you ask them for names and phone numbers of residents' relatives. The care-centre staff must abide by the *Freedom of Information and Protection of Privacy Act* and will not release any personal information.

In my opinion, there is nothing wrong with striking up a friendly conversation with others while you are touring a property. Introduce yourself and your parent as a potential new resident and casually ask for opinions. When it comes to choosing a long-term care facility for your parent, you can never ask too many questions. Remember, there are no foolish questions and, chances are, one question will naturally lead to the next. If you do not understand an answer or feel you have received an incomplete reply, press for more information.

If you have no idea of where or how to begin searching for a long-term care centre, ask for recommendations from others. Your family physician, hospital social workers, seniors' associations, and friends who are also caregivers can all be excellent sources of information.

If you are comparing different sites, take a notepad with you on each trip to record your thoughts and observations. You may also want to make a few photocopies of the Researching Long-Term Care Facilities worksheet found at the back of this book so you have a worksheet for each site tour. Rate each point from one to five (where "one" is poor and "five" is excellent). You can note any additional comments on the reverse side of the sheet. If you feel uncomfortable taking notes as you tour each building, do so immediately afterward so nothing will be forgotten.

You can also carry along a small, handheld tape recorder to verbally record any thoughts you may have. As with note taking, feel free to record your private thoughts when you are back in your car. It is best to do this immediately after you leave when your thoughts remain fresh. With the accumulated completed facility paper reports, I would highly recommend that you keep them together — perhaps in a binder or file folder.

Should you have the choice when it comes to where to move your parent (e.g., you may have only one long-term care facility in your area that is appropriate), weigh the alternatives carefully. Ensure that you are placing your parent in proper care, which is dependent on his or her needs. If your parent is able to tour the facilities with you and give you an opinion, by all means get his or her input. However, if your parent is unable to accompany you or share coherent thoughts, ask yourself if he or she would be pleased with the accommodations.

The information and questions in the following sections will help you and your parent decide if a facility is the right choice.

2.1 Location

Location can definitely be important for both you and your parent. Before we moved Dad into continuing care, he and my mother lived at a senior's residence, which offered independent living (e.g., meals, laundry service, and medication reminders were available; however, residents were not required to use these services). One of the beauties of this property was its close proximity to our city's scenic river valley. When Dad was still mobile, I accompanied him for many walks along the valley paths. An avid and strong hiker in his younger years, Dad still kept up a great pace and obviously enjoyed stretching his legs.

You should carefully evaluate the location of the building:

- Is it a suitable location for you to visit your parent?
- Will it be convenient for you to take your parent on regular outings (e.g., church services)?
- Is the property close to a hospital?
- Is the building in a safe neighbourhood for older people?
- Are stores for groceries, prescriptions, or other regular essentials; doctor's offices; banks; coffee shops; or parks located nearby?
- Is there a passenger loading and unloading zone located in front of the property's front door? You should be able to park there temporarily when picking up or dropping off your parent. An additional bonus would be a loading zone that is sheltered to protect your parent from bad weather such as rain or snow.

Another question to consider is whether there is ample visitor parking. What I had initially perceived to be a large parking lot at my father's facility proved to fill up quite quickly as both care staff and visiting family members parked there. If you do not drive, you will have to find out about access by public transit. What is the scheduling? When my father was alive, I wasn't driving. My weekly trips via the bus were on Sunday afternoons when I encountered reduced transit service.

2.2 Maintenance and cleanliness

Check the appearance and condition of the building. Ask yourself the following questions to ascertain the conscientiousness of the building's cleaning and maintenance staff:

- If you are visiting in the winter, are the sidewalks cleared of snow and ice?
- In summer, glance at the outside grass; is it neatly trimmed?
- Are there cracks in the sidewalks?
- Could the exterior walls use a fresh coat of paint?
- Is the facility clean and well lit?
- How thorough is the janitorial or housekeeping staff?
- Are spills mopped up immediately or left ignored?

2.3 Care staff interactions with others

Observe the interaction between care staff and residents. You want to make sure that your loved one will be properly taken care of and that he or she will feel welcome in the facility, so ask yourself the following questions:

- As you enter each facility, do you feel welcomed?
- Is there a general office to which family members can report?
- Are you greeted immediately?
- Is the staff friendly? Did at least one staff member smile and say "hello" to you?
- Do the staff respond promptly to the residents' needs?
- While the staff may not have the time to mingle with the residents, is there acknowledgement at some level (perhaps a warm smile or greeting)?
- Do staff call residents by their first names?
- How qualified are the care staff? Remember that the number of staff can be reduced in the evenings or overnight as a cost-saving measure.

- Do the residents interact well with each other?
- Is the staff working or chatting amongst themselves?
- What is the level of care available and the ratio of care staff to residents?
- Are there any restrictions to when family caregivers can visit?

2.4 Additional services

Take note of any additional services available for residents within the building:

- Are there hairdressing and nail-care services onsite?
- Does the facility offer physiotherapy?
- If your parent is of a religious faith, does the centre cater to various denominations? If so, how? Is there a chapel onsite?
- What other activities are available and how often are these planned? Will your parent find these activities enjoyable and stimulating?
- Are the residents encouraged to move around independently?
- Is there a sunroom or patio?
- Is there a separate, well-vented room for residents who smoke?
- Are care meetings between family and facility staff routinely scheduled? These are excellent opportunities for family caregivers to be updated on their parent's health as well as to ask any pressing questions.
- Is extended care available, if need be?
- Can a senior be transferred within the same facility to receive specialized assistance?

2.5 Residents' rooms

View your parent's potential room. Consider the size, shape, and location of this room within the building. Some things to consider when viewing the room include the following:

- Window placement and accessibility: Your parent may find an eastern exposure pleasing for the morning sunrise. Can the window be opened? Depending on your parent's mental awareness, an open window could pose a risk; however, a warm summer's breeze blowing through the room or the laughter of children playing nearby can be very pleasant and therapeutic. If your parent is confined to a bed, is the window still close enough to offer a view outside?

- Can the bed be moved or adjusted for additional comfort?
- How much space is available for additional furnishings? What in the way of additional furnishings can be brought in?
- Will this room be shared with another resident? If so, how is the room divided?
- Are there any restrictive columns/pillars?
- Is the bathroom shared or independent?
- How much closet space is provided?
- Will the temperature in the room be either too warm or too cold for your parent?

With my father's lifelong connection with books, my family supplied him with a small bookcase and asked the facility's maintenance staff to install some wheels on the bottom. Even when the shelves were fully laden with titles, it was still easy enough to roll the bookcase away from the wall for ease of cleaning.

With Dad's room, curtains around each bed provided the only separation from his roommate. While more privacy would have been nice, it was not the biggest concern. Though your parent's comfort and preferences are important, finding the perfect set of circumstances is rare. Be prepared to compromise or prioritize, but if something is very important to your parent, do what you can to help accomodate his or her preference — it may change his or her experiences in a facility dramatically.

2.6 Meals

If possible, schedule your tour around the residents' mealtime. Doing so will help you find answers to the following questions:

- What is offered for meals?
- How is the food served to residents?
- Is the menu varied and appealing?
- Can the facility's kitchen accommodate for any menu preferences, food allergies, or diet requirements?
- If your parent is a strict vegetarian, will the staff prepare nutritious meals and offer variety for this type of diet?

- If your parent cannot hold cutlery tightly or chew food properly, can assistance be provided (e.g., can food be chopped, diced, or mashed)?

If possible, sample the food yourself to ensure nutritional value, proper serving temperature, and good taste. Residents in long-term care centres are frequently offered a standard meal, so don't assume that a fresh salad can be prepared or that a substitution can be made.

2.7 Cost and subsidization

One of the most pressing topics you may have is cost and subsidization. You will need to find out what the cost is for the care and ascertain if there are any hidden costs involved. The flat fee that your parent is paying for care may only cover the basic necessities; typically, anything "extra" will cost extra.

You will also need to check with your parent's health-insurance provider to see if the costs can be subsidized. Remember, while you will want the best care for your loved one, it can be expensive. Ongoing medical treatment may be necessary; without insurance, you or your loved one will be incurring much of the cost.

In my father's case, his long-term care centre offered sliding scale payments based on income. Those residents who could pay more were expected to do so; proof of a resident's income, of course, had to be provided.

2.8 Safety

Safety is an important topic to consider when it comes to the care of your loved one:

- When was the building last inspected?
- If there is an elevator, when was this last serviced?
- How often are building and elevator inspections scheduled?
- What is the emergency evacuation procedure? (Although my father and other residents were on the third floor of a long-term care centre, I was assured that they would be ushered down a flight of stairs. In remembering many of the residents here were confined to wheelchairs and were cognitively impaired, I now wonder how effectively this could have been carried out.)
- Does the centre have emergency lighting in case of a power outage?

- Are resident medications and toxic cleaning supplies safely locked up and out of reach of those who may be confused?
- Is the building well lit?
- Are there automatic sensors that trigger outside lights at night when someone is approaching?
- Is the main entry brightly lit (this can provide additional safety and security to a resident coming home in the evening)?

3. MOVING YOUR PARENT

When the time comes to relocate your parent to a new facility or long-term care, you have a couple of choices. You can either hire professional movers or do it yourself. With a great deal already on a caregiver's plate, there is a lot to be said for the convenience of hired help; however, you must be careful with how you choose to move your parent's belongings. If you have the lead time, start calling around a month or two in advance. Create a spreadsheet to record information and compare services. Find out if the company is bonded and ask for references. Will the company guarantee the move and reimburse you for any damaged goods?

For a previous move of my own, I found a company that subcontracted movers. Essentially, the moving staff created their own company and purchased their own truck. I liked this arrangement as I thought the movers would take greater care with transporting goods.

When moving my parents from Victoria to Alberta, my sisters and I also found a professional packing company to help us. Our parents' belongings were carefully packed and shipped to us. Of course, there was an extra expense for this service; however, paying for this was justified as it saved my sisters and I from the flights necessary and the time required to complete this massive job. As independent operators, this packing company also saved us a lot of emotional baggage. Consider how draining it would be to sort through your own parent's belongings.

If you prefer to tackle your parent's move yourself, expect an enormous job — especially if your parents live at a distance from you. As every situation is different, I cannot advise as to how much lead time you should allow; however, you can, and should, expect delays. This is Murphy's Law, which states that "anything that can go wrong, will go wrong." The following list should help you get organized and focus on what needs to be done.

- Gather ample, sturdy boxes for packing. Smaller boxes with handles are better to use so that you don't overpack and make them too heavy to carry. You can find boxes at your grocery store, place of work, liquor stores, and bookstores. Start collecting these boxes well in advance; the best time to check the businesses for boxes is about mid-month to avoid the last-minute rush of other movers. Try to get similar shapes of boxes so they will stack easier; remember to place heavier boxes at the bottom of each pile.

- Acquire packing tape and a black felt pen for marking contents and room destinations on the outside of the boxes.

- Ensure all packing is completed before moving day. Pile all your boxes close to the front door for quick and easy access.

- Donate, delegate, and discard. Downsizing is often necessary when moving an individual into long-term care, so you will need to find new homes for collectibles. If possible, donate extra clothing to a homeless shelter (call to ask if they have a pick-up service available). Donate the extra television set to a friend who is just taking possession of a new condo. Difficult as this may be, consider discarding anything that is simply no longer needed.

- Call to rent a moving truck at least a few weeks in advance. If you are planning to relocate your parent at the end of the month, know that this time is popular for many other people to move as well.

- Double-check that your moving truck includes a moving dolly, plenty of furniture blankets, and a loading ramp.

- Book off elevators, if necessary (at both your departure point and end destination).

- Map your trip to make the best use of time. Consider whether it would be easier to move your parent first and then deliver excess items to a storage facility, or vice versa. Also consider traffic patterns to avoid any rush-hour traffic. Are there any low-clearance bridges that will be too restrictive for a large moving truck?

- Choose someone who is comfortable driving the moving truck (the truck rental company may insist that the driver be the individual signing the rental contract). If you are uneasy about driving anything bigger than your own vehicle, take quieter streets to your destination.

- Enlist another driver to park his or her vehicle and at your destination hold a good space until you arrive with the truck.

- Be prepared for emotional challenges. Moving your parent into long-term care is not easy. When I helped to move Dad, I was hit hard on moving day by the stark reality that he wasn't going to get better.

- Consider the expenses involved with long-term paid storage of parental items. If you can't find a home for your parent's chesterfield, or can't bear to part with something, the option of storing this may seem quite appealing. Make sure this option is financially viable for you and your family.

- Try not to adopt extra items yourself. While I have taken a few parental belongings to help furnish my home and to remind me of my parents, I simply do not have the additional storage room needed for bigger items. Turning your garage or extra bedroom into a storage locker is not ideal either; you will be constantly reminded of everything, making healing all the more difficult. Consider a senior's moving/downsizing service to help limit clutter.

- Try to get the move done as quickly and smoothly as possible. This will allow your parent more "settling in" time in his or her new home. Doing this also allows you to return to a calmer life sooner.

- Schedule your move during a quieter time at the new facility. The disruption of you carrying boxes in may confuse other residents.

- Check with facility maintenance staff to see if additional storage space can be provided for your parent. My father's room was not big, so, after we moved him in, we were successful in having a shelf screwed into the wall. This provided extra room for family photographs, books, and other possessions.

- Exercise caution with what you move into your parent's new home. I was warned by Dad's facility staff that other residents may, unknowingly, pick up other's belongings and move them elsewhere. It could take months to find something. You don't want to risk losing a family heirloom. You may want to mark items with your loved one's name for future identification, if needed. Use a permanent marker.

- Confirm with facility staff what you can bring for your parent. A bookshelf stereo system or portable television may seem like an exceptionally good idea; however, neither may be allowed.

- Provide a proper wardrobe for your parent in long-term care. Looking good is one thing; however, clothes must be sensible. Considering a senior's reduced mobility and flexibility, shirts and sweaters should be buttoned or zippered, rather than pulled on over the head. Keep nightclothes simple; for example, nightgowns should not be layered but more formal, and flannel will provide warmth in the winter. As care staff frequently clothe residents, fasteners should be simple. On the suggestion of my father's care staff, I purposefully bought him a few shirts that were one size too large. The extra room made it far easier for a nurse to dress and disrobe Dad. Velcro straps provide an excellent alternative to standard shoelaces. Supply pants with stretch waists to allow for increased comfort. Belts can chafe and may be difficult to undo in times of personal emergencies. Professional or office attire may have been necessary in your parent's working years; however, ties and high-heeled shoes are unnecessary in long-term care. Unless you are offering to launder your parent's clothes, ensure that everything is easy care.

Treat yourself following the move. Recognize your accomplishment by going out for dinner or doing something special. Trust me, you will have earned it!

4. WHEN YOUR PARENT CAN NO LONGER DRIVE

A person's vehicle can provide tremendous freedom and independence. A senior with reduced vision, hearing, or reflexes behind a steering wheel can easily turn that vehicle into a deadly missile. After a lifetime of regular driving, however, a senior may not readily hand over the keys or admit that there is a potential risk. The convenience and appeal of driving can be great.

My sisters and I discussed the driving issue at length and decided that the best route to take with our parents was to show our joint concern. This was not a time to offer our help, but to insist. Together, we approached Mom and Dad, voiced our worry, and were successful at convincing our parents to give up the car keys. While it was a sad day when I accompanied Mom back to the auto dealer to sell her car, I was also very relieved.

Should your parent not be convinced, another option for taking away the car keys is to work with a family physician. Begin by booking an appointment for your parent — even on the premise of an annual check-up or a prescription refill. Prior to visiting the doctor, call the doctor's office and explain your situation in more detail. If you cannot speak to the doctor directly, share your concerns with the receptionist to relay to the doctor. When you do bring your parent for the examination, the doctor can now address the subject of driving and can urge parking the car permanently. Sad as it may seem, a parent will often heed the advice of a physician over similar advice from a family member.

Expect some disgruntled days and parental backlash. Note that having a car taken away can be humiliating. Now is the time to introduce your loved one to other means of transportation such as public transit, taxis, and seniors' driving services, as well as family and friends. A senior can still get around quite well and be far safer with the alternative transportation. Depending on your loved one's response, now may also be the time to create some make-work projects to help him or her feel needed and valued. As an example, a good friend of mine purposefully snapped a home furnace wire so that her dad could have something to fix. This may seem a little extreme to you, but it worked!

After your parent relinquishes the car keys, you will be called on to run more errands and provide shuttle service. If you drive a four-door model of car, this is better because they are far easier to get in and out of than compacts. Avoid any vehicle requiring a high step to climb in; your parent will not be as supple as in younger years. Also, a car with a large trunk or storage compartment (e.g., a station wagon) is perfect for carrying wheelchairs or scooters.

If appropriate, you may also want to obtain a disabled parking pass to hang from your vehicle's mirror. With one of these visible, you will be allowed to use reserved parking spots closer to building door entrances making it a shorter walk for your parent.

At the back of this book, you will find a Driving Safety Checklist that will help you evaluate your parent's level of driving capability.

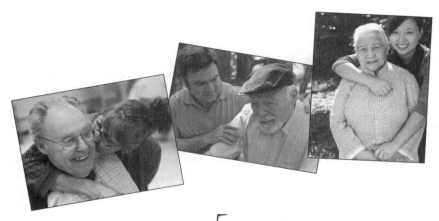

5
ORGANIZING YOUR
PARENT'S DOCUMENTS

"You can delegate authority, but not responsibility."

STEPHEN W. COMISKEY

Taking control of your parent's personal matters has to be one of the most challenging areas for a family caregiver. It is important that you keep the related documents safe and organized. It is also important for you to understand what these documents mean.

1. KEEP THE DOCUMENTS ORGANIZED

While you are organizing the paperwork, collect contact information for all of your parent's service providers (i.e., doctor, banker, financial planner, lawyer, real estate agent, etc.). Do not just carelessly stack business cards on the kitchen counter or toss them into a drawer; find a better means of retaining these so they will not get lost. I purchased a small business card holder (you can find these at any office supply store) to keep these secure. Another option is to attach a cork bulletin board to your wall and to pin your collected cards to it. When the bulletin board is placed by your home telephone, you can have all of your caregiving contacts handy; however, if you need to call or check in with someone when you are away from home, this is not quite as convenient. Your collection of caregiving business cards should not be excessive, but keeping these all in one place will keep you better organized.

Ensure you store your business card holder in a safe place such as inside a desk drawer instead of on top of your kitchen counter, where it could get lost with the daily mail. If you have a cellular telephone, take a few minutes to program the corresponding phone numbers into its memory. Many cellular phones also allow you to record additional contact information including email addresses and alternate phone numbers. You are doing yourself a favour by programming this information into your phone because you never know if, and when, you may need it when you are away from home.

If you do not do so already, I also strongly encourage you to create an effective and efficient filing system. As a caregiver, you will accumulate ample paperwork and will need to store it. Until I realized I had to become better organized, I had papers and notes to myself strewn about my home. With realizing this system was not highly effective, I purchased a small two-drawer filing cabinet and used different coloured file folders to keep information easily accessible. I'm a very visual person, so keeping the files colour-coded meant I could immediately pluck out what I needed, such as my green file for banking, my yellow file for medical, and so on.

In addition to long-term storage of documents, you may also want to create a shorter-term filing system of what needs to be done on a weekly basis. Using an accordion file, label each pocket with the days of the week. Slide your personal notes into each pocket; for example, mom's doctor's appointment on Tuesday, her haircut on Thursday, and medication pick-up on Friday. If you miss an appointment, or if it gets rescheduled for any reason, it is simple to transfer the note into another daily pocket or keep it where it is for the same time next week.

You can also note these appointments in a dayplanner; however, I found that page space was limited. If you choose to do this, look for a dayplanner with a one page per day layout, which will give you more room to write in multiple appointments. I also paper clipped or stapled any accompanying information required (e.g., a business card with an office address, a dry-cleaning receipt, or a prescription notice to be refilled) to the specific page, which is a practice I still follow today.

You may prefer another means of organization such as a dry-erase board on your wall to note any upcoming appointments. Maybe you work better with an in-and-out basket to filter jobs requiring your attention and jobs which have been completed. For best results, choose the system that is right for you. Filing systems are not iron-clad; these can be adopted and streamlined as needed.

While you will be collecting receipts, bills, and bank statements in your parent's name, do not hang on to such documents needlessly. This not only creates a mountain of paperwork, it also becomes a risk for identity theft. Buy a home shredder. Spend a few more dollars on it to ensure better quality. My first home shredder was less expensive and quickly proved incapable of handling the increased load. Personally, I like the heavier-duty shredders that can shred credit cards and staples as well as handle multiple sheets of paper at one time. If your shredding does get out of hand, look for a mobile shredding company in your city or town. In my area, a fully equipped shredding truck will come to my door for document destruction. Maybe your banker, accountant, or lawyer could be convinced to provide safe disposal? Do not overlook community organizations either; for example, the Alberta Motor Association schedules free public-shredding events annually.

To keep yourself organized, ensure you complete the Caregiver's Document Worksheet, Medical History Log, and Medication Log located at the end of this book.

2. UNDERSTANDING THE IMPORTANT DOCUMENTS

It is not enough for you to know where your parent's important documents are — you must also understand what the documents are about. It upset me greatly to read both my parents' living wills (also known as advance directives). These are documents that outline a person's care and treatment preferences, should he or she be unable to share this information, for any reason. Even though I was uncomfortable reading this information, my knowing, valuing, and accepting my parents' final wishes was vital. I may have been asked by a doctor at any time to be a spokesperson for either my mother or father. I know that both of my parents did not wish to be kept alive simply for the sake of continuing to live. My parents both deeply respected quality of life and felt if they could not "meaningfully contribute" in some manner, neither of them wanted to be kept alive via medical or artificial means. While the subject weighed heavily on me many times, I was fortunately never called on to make one of life's most difficult decisions. I truly do not know if I ever could have done this.

2.1 Your parent's will

It is important to know where your parent's will is located. It could be stored with your parent's lawyer at his or her legal firm or it could be somewhere in your parent's home. You will need to find out if it is up-to-date and properly witnessed. Ascertain whether your parent was of sound mind when he or she signed it. Wills can be changed and updated for any number of reasons (e.g., your parent may have remarried or divorced, a beneficiary has died, or the value of the estate has substantially improved or worsened).

It is vital that you have access to the most current, properly-executed version of your parent's will, as this will void any earlier wills that have been created. If changes are desired or necessary with this document, it will be best to have a completely new will created (rather than including handwritten notes or striking out sections of text). If you cannot find your parent's will or if it simply does not exist, encourage your parent to consult a lawyer that specializes in wills to have one created as soon as possible.

Many caregivers use safety deposit boxes to lock away the important documents; however, you could also invest in a small, fireproof home safe — you can often find a suitable model at any office supply or hardware store. You can also use the safety deposit box or safe to store other important paperwork including your parent's personal medical records, insurance coverage, birth certificate, passport, home ownership papers, and health-care card number. For the sake of convenience, you can use your safe or safety deposit box to keep other items safe such as extra parental house or car keys.

2.2 Trusteeship and guardianship

When it comes to minding your parental matters, you may do so either voluntarily or by legal appointment as either guardian or trustee, or both. These two terms can be easily confused. A guardian will become responsible for a dependent adult's lifestyle choices (e.g., where he or she lives and who can care for him or her). A trustee will become responsible for a dependent adult's financial matters (e.g., collecting income tax slips, making investment decisions, and accounting for purchases made using the dependent adult's own money).

As guardian or trustee, you will receive official court-issued orders. You will need to distribute these orders to others for them to retain in their files — for instance, such as one to your parent's doctor's office, your parent's bank, your parent's long-term care centre, etc.

Guardianship and trusteeship are very different levels of care so it is vital to differentiate between them. You may learn at the wrong time that you do not have the authority to make a key decision. Both guardians and trustees must be caring and conscientious, yet a trustee must also be completely financially trustworthy, ethical, and hold high integrity. Your parents will frequently appoint their own trustees (commonly, the eldest child); however, such decisions can be legally overturned if necessary. Keep in mind that overturning a trusteeship can be a complicated (not to mention potentially thorny) matter; proceed with this action only when there is no other recourse.

A power of attorney is associated with both guardianship and trusteeship. The power of attorney is an official court document designating the individual appointed. It is important to distinguish between the different types of power of attorney; for instance, there is a power of attorney for property as well as a power of attorney for personal care. Note that each province and territory has different names for each of these orders, so you may need to talk to a lawyer to find out what you need specifically for your parent's situation.

You may be more familiar with the term "enduring power of attorney." With this type of document, the designated appointee can make financial decisions for the incapable adult. A power of attorney for personal care is used by the appointee to oversee daily living for the senior so the appointed person can decide on accommodation, care providers, and medical treatments.

There are many good books that specifically discuss the topics of guardianship and trusteeship, so I will not launch into extensive details differentiating between them here. I must stress, however, that minding the parental finances can be a highly contentious issue because each family member may raise solid points or strong arguments as to how to allocate funds. There may be emotional baggage attached to money matters as well. Like it or not, greed (whether subconscious or conscious), can also become a motivating factor for some family members. A simple matter like contributing to a mutual fund or donating to a charity on your parent's behalf can become a highly flammable argument amongst family members.

If you are an only child, you will not have such obvious opposition, but you will also not have the benefit of having a sibling's perspective. With multiple family caregivers, the safest way to approach these conversations is openly. Share all the relevant information. Is there any information or a recommendation from an unbiased subject matter expert to consider? Allow each person a chance to completely air his or her opinions. Do not interrupt any speakers; write down any questions you have, and ask your questions after the speaker has finished. Watch your own body language as well; when crossing your arms across your own chest, you are resisting. Voting can help ease matters. If a stalemate still exists, bring in an outside negotiator. If your parent cannot advise for any reason (e.g., cognitive impairment or inability to speak), try to make your decisions as to how your parent would react. If a situation poses risk, for example and you know that your parent was not a risk taker, look at other avenues. Ask yourself, "What would Mom/Dad have done in this situation?"

When it comes to applying for trusteeship or guardianship, a lawyer is the common choice for help. With a little digging, you may find assistance with this paperwork elsewhere. My sisters and I were pleasantly surprised when we discovered a local seniors' agency that included a guardianship department. The qualified staff worked with visitors to decipher the documentation and complete the necessary forms. The one disadvantage was that family members and friends applying for guardianship would be called on to serve the papers personally; however, doing this was available at a fraction of the cost of a high-priced lawyer.

The responsibilities of both guardians and trustees can be enormous and may be too much for one person to handle. My older sister and I served as co-guardians and co-trustees for Dad — she was the primary and I was the alternate. This arrangement proved to be useful on several occasions when my older sister was out of town and had to assign the authority over to me. Mind you, she did have to write a letter each time to temporarily provide me the authority necessary. Having two of us working together also helped elsewhere — I think specifically of those times when we were called on to create a regular financial spreadsheet showing our financial decisions for Dad, which held us accountable. Admittedly, math is neither of our strongest points. Therefore, having two of us working on it provided both encouragement and motivation to get the job done. In the back of this book you will find a Caregiver's Financial Expenses Log to help you stay organized.

It is entirely possible that a dependent adult may not have a guardian or trustee appointed. He or she may have never made that decision, the initial appointee may have become sick or died, or the initial appointee may have refused the appointment. In such cases, when no one is available or willing to manage the senior's affairs, you can contact your closest Office of the Public Guardian or Office of the Public Trustee to make alternate arrangements. These offices can step in and safeguard dependent adults by managing their finances, making decisions about personal care, choosing treatment options, and so on.

To learn more, I recommend you read the book entitled *Protect Your Elderly Parents: Become Your Parents' Guardian or Trustee,* also published by Self-Counsel Press. Written by Lynne Butler, this book is a superb guideline for where to start, what to expect, what to watch out for, and how to best help your parent by taking on these roles.

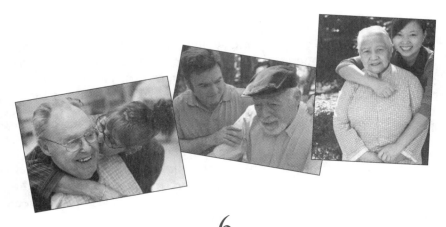

6
VISITING DAY

"It's not about how much time you spend together; it's what you do with the time you do spend together."

UNKNOWN

How often you visit your parent in long-term care is your choice; however, seeing him or her as often as possible is best, in my opinion. Hard as it may seem to admit, your parent may not have long to live and the final months will be your last chance to spend time with your parent. While long-term care centres are becoming more welcoming, you may remain uncomfortable with visiting. Despite this, your parent can still benefit from the socialization — and so can you.

Should you feel uneasy about visiting, consider doing so for the benefit of your parent. Imagine if you were confined to an institution or, worse yet, a hospital bed where you could not move; think of how welcome a friendly face would be. Would your mood not dramatically improve? If nothing more, you could sit beside a hospital bed and hold your loved one's hand to share love. Even after Dad lost his ability to speak, I was able to do this and maintain a connection with him.

A good friend of mine once shared with me that he chose not to visit his grandmother in long-term care as it was simply too painful for him to see her in that condition. She lived for two more years and he now accepts that not going to see her was a huge mistake on his part.

Another reason to visit is being able to personally monitor the daily care regimen of your loved one. While I held the utmost respect for my father's care staff, seeing the care staff and how they worked provided me with increased peace of mind. Try to mix up your visiting times to keep care staff on their toes. Through regular visits, you can also become more involved with your parent's care.

1. ACTIVITIES TO DO WITH YOUR LOVED ONE

Your loved one's medical condition will, of course, largely determine what you can do with him or her and when. I count my blessings that Dad remained mostly mobile until the end so that we could take our weekly walks. When it comes to planning activities with your loved one, think of what your parent previously enjoyed:

- Can you take him or her outside in a wheelchair to enjoy some fresh air and sunshine?
- Can you read a story out loud to him or her?
- Can you watch a travel video featuring a favourite destination?
- Can you listen to music or join a singalong?
- Can you bring in your cat or dog to share some unconditional love?

When it comes to possible activities, think outside the box too. A neighbour of my father's in long-term care had his room walls plastered, from floor to ceiling, with family photographs. This way, he was continually surrounded by familiar faces and sights.

Can you enlist your loved one's help with folding laundry? This suggestion may seem a little strange; however, I learned that even when the mind has forgotten, an individual with Alzheimer's disease can still perform routine functions with his or her hands. You could bring in a laundry basket of towels and ask your parent to help you fold these. When the basket is done, explain that you are putting them away and leave the room for a few minutes. While you are gone, toss the towels around and return with "another load."

Some other creative ideas for your visit could include the following:

- Pack a picnic and include a brightly coloured picnic blanket.
- Play a simple card game.
- Roll out a practice putting green (use a plastic golf club).
- Try bowling with a plastic bowling ball and pins.
- Plant or tend to flowers inside your parent's room.

- Write joint letters to family and friends.
- Finger paint.
- Enlist your parent's help with stuffing and sealing card envelopes prior to Christmas.

Dad's facility staff also organized regular field trips for residents where family members could come along. Make the effort to participate these field trips; they will make good memories for both you and your parent.

Keep in mind not just activities, but other comforts your loved one might not have access to within the facility. With my father always being a great fan of coffee, I began the habit of stopping by a coffee shop on my trip over to see him, to pick up either an iced or steaming cup of coffee — season dependent. It gave me great joy to watch Dad eagerly clasp the cup with his wrinkled hands, gulp down the drink, and smile.

Another recommendation for visiting day is to interview your parent. Use a small tape recorder — don't forget the extra batteries, just in case — and a list of questions to ask about earlier years. While I never had the opportunity to do this with my own parents, I was once, as a freelance writer, hired by two daughters to visit and question their father. For this, I used a digital recorder; the sound quality was excellent and there were no cassette tapes to fumble with during the interview.

Try to perform the interview in a smaller, distraction-free room. A low ceiling reduces recording echoes. If possible, shut the door to outside noise. Understand that your parent may speak quietly, so try to situate the recorder closer to his or her mouth without being obtrusive. Identify the best times of day to interview your parent. Is Mom or Dad more alert in the morning, for example? If so, you will likely get more detailed and complete answers to your questions at this time. Exercise patience here as you may hear the same stories repeated and, depending on your loved one's memory, facts may change.

When quizzing, you can help both yourself and your parent by noting down where you "left off" so you can easily prompt your parent with a reminder of what you were talking about previously. You can also bring a list of prepared questions to fill in during possible lulls in your conversation. When it comes to asking questions, don't be shy! Your parent may be flattered to be asked about his or her earlier life. With having these recordings, you will also have these stories for future generations.

Common games can be adapted for those in wheelchairs. Can your parent toss a sponge dart, play a game of cards, or participate in lawn bowling? One of the most creative recommendations I learned of was wheelchair dancing. Look for a dance school offering joint classes so that you and your parent can take part together. While your loved one may be restricted to a wheelchair, you should assess activities depending on what he or she *can* do rather than what he or she *cannot* do.

You can always just talk with your parent. Although your parent is in long-term care and may seem a shadow of who he or she once was, this is still the same person who loved you, cared for you, and counselled you through your previous life's trials and tribulations. If you cannot generate any further dialogue past asking, "How are you feeling today?" (followed by an uncomfortable silence) then come prepared. There are several ways to do this.

Prior to visiting, you could slide a few old family photos in your pocket; if these are pictures of family trips, all the better. When you arrive, you can show these to your loved one with a verbal prompt such as, "I found these photos of our vacation to Disneyland. Wasn't that a fun time?" Aging brains may still remember such special family times fondly. Try doing this and you could be rewarded with plenty of smiles and laughter. Although I heard Dad's story of how Cattle Point (a visitor's site in Victoria, British Columbia) was named more times than I care to remember, there are still times when I would like to hear him recount it once more. I learned with my father that it was more important to talk to him when I could. Be understanding, patient, and forgiving if your parent does not remember all the exact trip details.

Another idea to generate discussion is to clip some magazine articles. You may want to avoid newspaper write-ups that report on current news, of which your parent may be unaware. While your parent may not admit this, he or she could be silently embarrassed about not knowing what is going on directly outside his or her home. Instead, choose stories of personal achievement or social values. Your prompt here could sound like this: "I have just read this incredible story of a blind man who climbed Mount Everest. Have you ever wanted to scale a mountain peak?" Ask your questions based on your parent's previous knowledge or interests. Keep your questions open-ended because these types of questions require a more extensive answer than a simple "yes" or "no." With a spirited conversation, your loved one will become more enthusiastic to share with you.

Because of seniors' reduced energy, keep your visits short and understand the difference between good (when your parent is lucid) and bad days. Try not to be disappointed or blame yourself if your parent was not coherent when you came to visit. This is not something you can take control or blame for. Instead, accept it and hope for a better day tomorrow. The better days can be magical.

2. FINDING THE BEST TIME TO VISIT

While family caregivers are often allowed 24-hour access to their loved one, you may have to adjust your visiting schedule to accommodate your parent. If he or she likes to take a regular mid-afternoon nap, this is probably not the best time to drop by. Personally, when I found Dad napping, I always let him sleep.

Mealtimes, when care staff are trying to feed residents, can be very hectic; your presence may be more of a hindrance than a help. If your parent has any regular appointments with care staff (e.g., haircut, pedicure, or physiotherapy treatment), you will want to find out the schedule so you don't come at those times. I learned that my father was bathed on Sundays, which was something I really couldn't (or didn't want to) interrupt! Ask your parent's care staff for recommendations as to the best visiting times.

For your best visiting experience, look for a private place where you and your parent can spend time together. Long-term care centres can be busy places and not usually conducive to quality, quiet family time. Is there a private visiting room onsite? If so, ensure this will be available at your scheduled time. If there is no such space available, why not make the recommendation to care centre management to incorporate such a room?

With our Sunday family dinners, we began by booking a small room on the third floor (we had to get our names in early in the week as this room proved to be popular). It was a simple matter to close the door to shut out most of the noise and commotion from outside. Unfortunately, the room proved to be quite cramped for our purposes so we eventually had to look elsewhere for a spot to dine with Dad.

3. CELEBRATING HOLIDAYS AND BIRTHDAYS

I strongly recommend visiting your parent on birthdays and holidays. These days can remain very significant for many people as they age. Don't come empty-handed. Bring along a birthday or Christmas present. Choosing something may seem difficult for someone in long-term care because you are not sure what the person may need or what will be suitable. Understand that your parent will be appreciative for any number of things — thinking practically here will be best. The following are a few ideas:

- Comforter for the bed. This will keep your parent warm at night and add a splash of colour to the room. Look for a bedspread that can be easily laundered.

- Slippers. Some warm and fuzzy footwear can be very much appreciated. Choose a form-fitting, rather than floppy, style for safer walking.

- Subscription for audiobooks. Aging eyes may not be able to read fine print anymore; however, your parent may still be still able to listen to and enjoy a good story.

- Rechargeable razor. Personal hygiene remains important for your parent while in long-term care. Cordless models of razors can be used anywhere, so your dad might use it while sitting on his bed or in a dining room chair. Empty the razor regularly to keep it operating smoothly. However, be sure to keep the razor tucked away out of sight or bring it with you on visiting day. In my father's unit, such smaller objects often could be mistakenly picked up by other residents and spirited away somewhere. You would be lucky if you could ever find these items again.

- Home-baked cookies. Who doesn't like to nibble a delectable treat? Watch out for food allergies, though, and don't bring more than your parent can reasonably eat in a short time. Although having a few "extra" cookies around for later may seem harmless, these may attract unwanted guests (e.g., bugs or rodents) into your parent's room. Be aware that even the smell of many food items (such as peanuts) can trigger allergic reactions. Even if your parent is likely to consume these quickly, you will want to check with the facility staff to see if there will be any potential problems.

- Holiday decorations. Share some seasonal merriment with a festive wreath. You can hang this in your parent's room or on the room door.

- Small bookshelf stereo. Ask facility staff first before bringing any radios or CD players because the sound may be disturbing to others. If allowed, your parent might enjoy listening to nostalgic CDs. If your parent will be operating the stereo, choose a model with larger controls or pre-programmable radio station buttons.

- Bathrobe. Choose a terrycloth style for increased warmth. As with all clothes supplied, make sure this can be easily laundered. While a coloured robe can add some brightness, the dyes may bleed and damage other clothing. To solve this problem, wash the new coloured robe in cold water a few times separately before giving it to your parent. Tie a couple of knots in the robe belt to attach this to the belt loops; by doing so, the robe's belt is less likely to go astray.

- Flowers. Brighten any room with a fresh bouquet of beautiful flowers. Not only will flowers colour a dull room, they smell wonderful and will also improve mood. Recipients of fresh flowers can become happier. Place these in a plastic vase to avoid accidental breakage. As with even small food items, the fragrance of flowers can cause unpleasant allergic reactions; be sure to confirm with facility staff what is safe to bring in to the facility.

- Massager. A little touch of heaven! As with the razor, look for one that can be operated without an electrical cord.

- Grandchildren's drawings. Invite youngsters to draw and colour a picture for you to take to your parent. Completed pictures can be taped onto a wall. A personal drawing can hold special significance for your loved one.

- Family photo album. Supply your parent with fresh pictures to look at.

Presents don't have to be material to be appreciated. Having the grandchildren visit and sing a rousing rendition of "Happy Birthday" or a holiday song should surely bring a smile to your parent's face.

While I urge you to visit on birthdays and other holidays throughout the year, one of the most difficult times to see a parent can be the winter holiday season. So much of this time of year focuses on the family being together; when you visit, family memories may resurface and remind you that things have changed. It is time for you to look at changing some old family traditions and creating new memories. Know that you can still keep some memories alive and involve your parent in the celebrations, even if he or she cannot join you in the way he or she used to.

One of my father's traditions was to read "'Twas the Night before Christmas." Maybe you will want to enlist another family member to employ the same traditions during your holiday celebration in commemoration.

The following are some suggestions as to how to make new memories while combining them with old traditions:

- Gather the family together and view collected photographs.
- String up holiday decorations.
- Share your stories; laugh and cry together. Doing so can be very therapeutic.
- Use your mom's old gravy bowl with your turkey dinner.
- Continue to send the regular holiday family letter to distant friends.
- Tour your city and view holiday displays.

Create a new decoration; for example, use a small photo of your parents, frame it, and make it festive. I learned that my father's care centre honoured previous residents with pictures. I took part in a festive ceremony where I strung Dad's photo from a tree branch. By hanging this picture from your tree at home, your parent will still be with you over the holidays, even when he or she cannot physically be there.

If you can, involve your mother or father in your own family celebrations away from the care facility. Remember that your parent may easily tire and a full day may prove to be too much to handle. With my father's Alzheimer's disease, he disliked sudden and loud sounds, which included his own excited grandchildren squealing with delight when they opened their Christmas presents. We found it necessary to shorten his visits. Try scheduling another activity for the grandchildren outside of your home (e.g., take them tobogganing or skating) so that your parent can enjoy some peace.

Depending on your parent's condition, perhaps she or he can still participate in an outdoor activity. While my father's mind was sliding, he remained in good physical shape in his later life. Knowing Dad's fondness for sport, we took him to a local ski hill but we were not sure of what to expect. We had Dad sized for rental boots, ski poles, and skis. While the hill paled in comparison to a mountain slope in Jasper or Banff, Dad, much to our delight, smoothly and confidently rode the T-bar up and swooped back down, carving huge turns in the snow.

With an extended visit to your home, whether over the winter holidays or any other time during the year, remember to pack an extra change of clothes for your parent or have clean clothes waiting in your closet. Should any emergencies arise, you will have something clean and dry for your parent to wear.

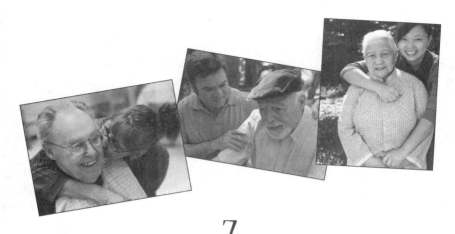

7

WORKING WITH OTHER FAMILY MEMBERS AND MAINTAINING HARMONY

"In time of test, family is best."

BURMESE PROVERB

When you and your siblings are all looking after your parents, expect some differences of opinion. You may not always agree on the same course of action. There will be mild skirmishes and more serious verbal battles. It's easy for one family member to get his or her feathers ruffled when opinions are not readily accepted.

If and when possible, you will want to remain on the same page with your siblings. Keeping things harmonious between siblings just makes perfect sense. It is far easier to work and live with someone when you agree. Furthermore, important caregiving decisions can be made far more quickly without delays.

Although with caregiving, maintaining peace within the family is easier said than done. Expect roadblocks or resistance from those closest to you. Everybody will feel that they have the best answer. For the benefit of all involved, try to keep an open mind and maintain clear lines of communication.

Caregiving can result in emotional and frustrating times. Your parent's health is failing and there may be little or nothing that can be done. Tempers can flare without warning over the smallest issues. This may relate back to an old emotional "button" which could somehow be important to an individual. Situations can easily be emotionally charged at times. A family caregiver has not only his or her past and present to deal with; he or she may be already anticipating a bleak or painful future in regards to his or her parent's condition.

Sad as it seems, we humans also like to be right about things. Knowing that we have made the proper decision makes us feel good; making that proper decision on behalf of someone else only increases our joy.

We often take offence to being challenged with our recommendations. Therefore, make your recommendations to your siblings softly. Tread lightly for the sake of your future relationships. Do not push your opinion onto others. Support your argument with solid facts ("I *think* we should do this" is not going to be enough). When you do make the proper decision regarding your parent's care, do not boast. Nobody will like to hear this. Try not to raise your voice because it often makes a listener immediately more defensive.

The best way to avoid an argument is by not starting one — although this can be unrealistic. Once an argument has begun, one of the most useful tools to deflate it is through active listening. It may be more important for the speaker to be heard than to actually win the verbal war. The speaker may be venting frustration at the situation that is not even intended for you. Therefore, remove distractions from the room, pay attention to the speaker, lean forward, and nod. Allow the speaker to fully vent without interruptions and then paraphrase for full clarity. Do not dismiss anything stated as not being important or harshly judge what has been said. If a point has been raised, it is important to the person who made the comment. If numerous points have been raised, ask the speaker to prioritize them in order of importance.

You will want to begin each familial conversation by saying something positive. It is human nature to get immediately self-protective or defensive when we feel we have been targeted as having made a mistake or being wrong. Therefore, open your meeting with a compliment rather than a comment. You may still face resistance; however, others will be more open to listening and dialoguing with you. Similarly, if you are providing feedback on another's point of view, do so carefully. Implement the "sandwich technique" of evaluating others. Begin with a positive affirmation or two, make your suggestion for improvement, and then finish with another positive statement. Communication will be far more pleasant.

Plan to keep your own family meetings brief. By being attentive to the clock, your conversations will become more productive. If a problem does not have to be addressed immediately, postpone conversation until a better time or take small steps toward resolving the issue. Using these approaches can often be far more effective than tackling the entire issue head-on. If you have ever made a New Year's resolution, you will know that you can become far more successful making a smaller promise, which makes the larger goal much more attainable. By stalling the discussions a day or so, everybody can return to the deliberating table with clearer heads.

Recognize the time of day. Arguing late at night is pointless because people are tired and need to sleep. Emotions and worry regarding getting up in the morning can run even higher at this time. It is unlikely that you will solve any problems when you are exhausted. In fact, you are not doing yourself or your loved one any favours by not getting some rest and returning to those issues the next day.

If your family has the benefit of time before a decision must be made, by all means, take as much as you need. One highly effective problem-resolution tool is to brainstorm possible answers and take a few days to mull these ideas over in one's mind. This often allows an individual to come back with a fresh, complete, and better perspective. For example, with my writing, I always appreciate having some "breathing time" before a project deadline. This allows me to put the project aside for a day or so and then return to it with an increased vigour.

If you and your siblings live apart, alternate these meetings between your homes. Doing so will provide more neutral ground and will level the playing field. Also, try to hold conversations in an open room without barriers (e.g., a desk or a coffee table) between you. You do not want to appear oppositional during these discussions. If you expect these discussions to become heated, appoint a moderator (someone who is mutually agreed on and respected) to help keep things under control.

If possible, assign someone as a secretary to take notes. This way you can distribute copies of what was said, and you can also review past conferences before proceeding, thus saving a great deal of time.

No matter what you speak of with your siblings, the most highly contentious issues surround your parent's will and any potential inheritances. Depending on individual circumstances, even the closest of siblings can bicker about this. The anticipated monies can drive a wedge between brothers and sisters — a wedge so large that it may temporarily, or even permanently, alienate and completely separate family members from ever speaking to each other in the future.

In my opinion, it is best for all monies to remain solely for the use of the senior until his or her final breath. If your parent is of sound mind and wants to gift some money to adult children, this is another matter. Should this occur, you may wish to document the transfer of funds for everybody's complete protection. Do not consider any early withdrawals or creative loans against those funds. Although you may well be looking at a sizable sum of money, remember to make sound financial decisions based on what your parent would choose to do. Reserve the majority of accumulated savings for future health needs. Remember, health care can be very pricey and one cannot possibly predict what expenses lie ahead.

When holding your family meetings, do not simply focus on the current issues. Look ahead. As with all caregiving issues, it is better to be proactive rather than reactive with your own discussions. By discussing anticipated problems amongst yourselves, you will be better prepared. By learning more about your parent's health condition, you will have a more complete understanding of the possible outcomes. If your parent, like my father, has Alzheimer's disease, know that a secured facility will be required at some time. Start investigating the housing options available. Will Mom or Dad require a motorized scooter? Will modifications be required at home? Do you need to clarify any of your parent's final requests? Please don't leave those decisions until the last minute or to chance. These are not easy conversations to begin; however, it is far better to make those necessary plans now rather than later. Reach out, research, and prepare.

Depending on the time you have and your family have, try to focus on fewer issues during your meetings. Less is more. By deliberating on just one or two caregiving challenges at a time, you will be better able to give each topic the utmost attention that it deserves.

Keep your conversations timely as well. For example, realistically you shouldn't have to discuss taxation issues until January or February. Are there more pressing matters that need you and your family's immediate attention? Devote your attention and energies where they are most needed.

Another book also published by Self-Counsel Press is *Estate Planning through Family Meetings*. This book can provide you with excellent advice on how to prepare and conduct family meetings to deal with these important issues.

1. WHAT TO DISCUSS DURING THE MEETINGS

What you speak about in your family meetings will, of course, be dependent on your own situation. The following sections outline a few key areas that will be specific to all caregivers and their family meetings.

1.1 Finances and banking

Knowing where your parent's money is coming from, how much is coming in, and where it is going requires some simple accounting. Draw up a balance sheet to confirm income and expenditures. Create a spreadsheet on your computer and save it to your desktop. This will make it easily accessible when you need to record another entry. Review your parent's financial situation regularly and go over this at the meetings, if necessary. There may be investments or mutual funds that will also need your attention so this should be a topic you discuss at the meeting.

Is there someone who is assigned to pay your parent's monthly bills? If so, that person may need to order new cheques or he or she may want to arrange for payments to be conveniently made through automatic withdrawal. Or the person might like to have a separate credit card so that he or she can buy items on behalf of your parent. (You can request additional credit cards and you should keep a minimal balance.)

1.2 Medications

What medications are currently prescribed to your parent? At the meeting you might want to discuss the medications and who is responsible for refilling the prescriptions. Also, decide who will make the doctor's appointment and who will take your parent to the doctor to get the refill for the prescription. Look into whether it is possible to set up an account with a medication delivery service, which are sometimes offered by pharmacies (thus saving you a trip).

You and your siblings may have noticed some nasty side effects your parent is having with medication. Decide what should be done about this, whether by talking to a doctor or a pharmacist.

1.3 Diet and personal care

You or your siblings may want to report to the others at the meeting about your parent's appetite. If your parent is having difficulty eating food, either by holding a utensil or with chewing or swallowing, then some options should be discussed. Can someone talk to the care staff about possible solutions to these types of situations?

Other issues may include how attentive care staff has been to your parent. At the meeting, you may want to discuss if anyone has noticed any questionable or irregular actions from the care staff. Also, you may have noticed actions from the care staff that you could commend, which should also be discussed. This may put your mind or a family member's mind more at ease, knowing the parent is being well taken care of in the care facility.

At the meeting you could include the topic of facility care inspection. Is there ignored ice on the front sidewalk of the care facility? Does a chair arm need tightening? Should a lightbulb in your parent's room be replaced? Is a toilet seat loose? Was the floor swept and mopped? If these areas are lacking the proper maintenance, then you need to discuss how to deal with these situations. When sharing these issues with care facility management, remain firm but calm. Also, follow the correct protocol — do you need to provide a written letter? (Keep a copy for your own files.) Or, do you need to discuss this at a monthly care meeting including facility managers and family caregivers?

1.4 Parental quality of life

Although a senior may be bed-bound in long-term care, he or she can still enjoy quality of life. Essentially, this means that he or she will be as healthy and happy as possible, be able to meaningfully contribute in some manner, and remain respected. Family caregivers should ensure that their loved one enjoys at least some level of personal independence (including personal privacy).

Some topics for your parent's quality of life may include sufficient supports such as inside and outside care staff, suitable medical equipment (e.g., wheelchairs), and necessary onsite services (e.g., physiotherapy, massage, exercise programs) in place and readily accessible.

Does your parent still have continued family relationships and social contact with friends? If not, can the group come to a decision at the meeting on what to do about your parent's lack of social situation? Are activities or recreational outings meaningful? Does your parent appear to be comfortable in the facility or are there obvious signs of discomfort or distress? Look for poor posture, restricted movement, and/or pained expressions as clues. If your parent cannot speak, it is even more vital that you speak for him or her.

1.5 Responsibilities

At the meetings, you might want to discuss whether everybody is still agreeable with their assigned caregiving duties. You might find that someone is experiencing unexpected difficulty with his or her role. If so, you may want to delegate these responsibilities to other family members, outside individuals, or service agencies so as to lighten the person's load. If everyone agrees, you could also rotate caregiving assignments amongst your siblings. This way, no one bears the burden of any excessive caregiving task for too long.

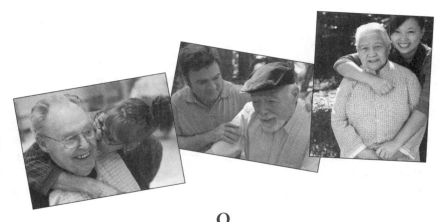

8
TAKING A BREAK

"To put the world in order, we must first put the nation in order; to put the nation in order, we must first put the family in order; to put the family in order, we must first cultivate our personal life; and to cultivate our personal life, we must first set our hearts right."

SAYS CONFUCIUS

When you are a caregiver, you must remember your own health and well-being. While the cliché of "taking care of yourself" has become very tired, you must think of your own needs in addition to thinking of those of your parent. You don't have to put yourself first; however, you should put yourself on an even keel to achieve much-needed balance. Doing so may sound selfish; yet, taking a personal break is anything but selfish. If you think of a car, the vehicle can only go so far without fuel and regular maintenance. To prevent yourself from overheating and requiring a major service overhaul, learn to walk away from caregiving occasionally. Book a personal tune-up. Aim to release yourself totally from your responsibilities (even on a short-term basis). You will come back stronger and more revitalized. Don't you always feel better after a good night's sleep? You simply cannot function forever without taking a rest.

1. DELEGATE SOME OF THE WORK

In the world of caregiving, "taking a personal break" is referred to as respite. There are various ways you can find respite, such as removing yourself from the situation in one way or another or delegating another individual to mind your parent temporarily.

As a caregiver, you do not have to try and handle everything yourself. You may feel like you have a responsibility to your parent, but with taking on too much, you are doing him or her more of a disservice. Overloading yourself is unwise and unsafe for both you and your loved one.

When looking back, and even looking at other current caregivers in my social circle, I now compare a caregiver's actions to a trip to a buffet; the caregiver will often persist with loading yet more food onto his or her own plate. Keep in mind, though, that the plate is only so large. You will either spill your food or drop the plate on the floor, as it becomes too heavy.

Wherever you may live, you can find individuals and services to help you. To help you identify these resources, please refer to the Your Circle of Caregiving worksheet, which is located at the back of this book. Obviously, in a larger city these will be more plentiful than in a small town. Ease up on your responsibilities. Delegate work to others. Let others help you. Be kind to yourself and never feel guilty or selfish for doing so.

2. SOCIALIZE AND PURSUE HOBBIES

For your own escape, socialize. Remember your friends; go meet someone for a cup of coffee and try and discuss matters other than your own caregiving experiences. Involve your friends when and wherever possible. Friends can be a tremendous support through offering either a sympathetic ear or a helping hand when you need it most.

How you can find personal respite is only limited to your own imagination. Other ways to take a break may include the following (in no particular order of preference):

- Pursue a hobby.
- Take up a new interest.
- Register in a class.

- Go for a walk. Don't use the excuse that it is too cold outside to not get some fresh air.
- Do something special with your significant other.
- Go to a concert.
- Book a massage.
- Wander through a museum or an art gallery.
- Volunteer.
- Go for a long drive.
- Rent a movie.
- Brew a pot of tea, and read a good book while sipping the tea.
- Book a weekend flight to a place such as Victoria: go whale watching, tour the Island on a double-decker bus, or relax in the scenic Inner Harbour.
- Watch a hockey or a baseball game, or some other sporting event.
- Head to your local mall and go shopping.
- Rake the leaves in your backyard.
- Clean your house.
- Organize a potluck supper with neighbours or friends.

As a freelance writer, I turned more to my craft for relief. You can write too — you do not have to be a professional — and nobody will ever see your journaling save for yourself unless you want them to. One beauty of writing is that you do not have to remain at home to write. Take a notebook and pen to the park. Take your laptop computer to the neighbourhood coffee shop. Try writing a letter to your parent to say what has not been said; while this may never be read, the action of journaling your innermost thoughts can be immensely healing.

3. JOIN A SUPPORT GROUP

While support groups aren't for everybody, they can provide an excellent means of respite for a caregiver. Support groups can vary in size and offer the opportunity for caregivers to share in a safe and supportive setting. For a support group novice, a smaller group will allow for more individual participation and is often less intimidating.

While talking in a support group can be beneficial, it is not obligatory; however, you are encouraged to contribute. Group attendees can just listen, learn, and leave feeling better about their own situations. Often, there is no charge to join a support group and participate.

Look for a support group offered at a convenient time and location for you. Remain open to the option of attending such a group with your sibling or other parent. Being in a sharing environment may encourage talking about difficult matters. If nothing else, the information and other stories shared can be absorbed by each family member present.

4. PAMPER YOURSELF

Pampering yourself occasionally is another form of caregiver respite. Give yourself a gift, because you certainly deserve it! These personal gifts do not have to be lavish or expensive. Of the many possible present ideas that exist, a caregiver will often most appreciate having personal time. Although it may sound or feel insensitive, get away from your parent for a while. Think back to the times when your parents would hire a babysitter for you when you were younger so they could slip out for a private evening together. They wanted, and needed, a break from parenting. In turning the tables, why do you not now deserve that same privilege?

Finding personal respite time over the holidays can become even more difficult. You may well want to curl up and forget about the holidays entirely while others are hanging decorations and being festive. With the heavy focus on the family at this time of year, it can become even easier to disregard or completely ignore your own needs. It is little wonder how caregivers can become even more discouraged during the holidays. Difficult as it may seem, try to remember the true spirit of the season.

For the past number of years, I have made it a point to do something non-commercial over the holidays — whether attending a concert or donating a frozen turkey to our local food bank. Whether this is a new custom or an adaptation of a former tradition, find something that works for you.

In addition, remember it will be okay to say "no" to an invitation. Just because it is the holidays, you are not obligated to give your time if you do not feel in a social mood. The same can be said for any other time throughout the year. I remember one year when I turned down an invitation to attend a work Christmas party. While this was a little unnerving to do, I simply explained that I was not up to celebrating. There was some confusion and resistance from my fellow workmates; however, when I further explained my reasoning, most accepted and understood my decision. Of course, the opposite can also be said. Toasting the season with friends may be just the ticket to chase away any caregiving doldrums. Do what feels right to you.

Enlist one of your caregiving team members to look after your parent and take some time for you. Once I learned to release the ever-tightening reins and take a breather myself, one of my favourite escapes was to a neighbourhood coffee shop. I would sip a tall coffee and read the daily newspaper. Even an hour of personal time away would refresh my mind and my mood and I would be ready to return to being an active caregiver. Whether planned or impromptu, caregiving breaks are vital for caregivers. Find an activity you enjoy and partake in it as often as possible.

If you prefer something more material as a present, treat yourself. Go out for dinner at a nice restaurant, buy yourself flowers, or book a professional massage. Any of these activities can be enjoyed throughout the year. Remember to stay within your own budget; if you cannot afford anything costly, even a small indulgence (e.g., chocolate or ice cream) can make you feel better.

When planning respite activities for yourself, I believe it is important to keep them independent from your family. It will do you little good to go out for dinner with your brother or sister as your topic of conversation could easily focus on what is happening with your parent.

5. FIND A DAY PROGRAM FOR YOUR PARENT

Explore other possibilities for respite. My sisters and I found a day program for Dad. Twice per week Dad would be picked up first thing in the morning and transported to a local seniors' centre. He would be occupied with games and other activities and then returned home later that afternoon. Doing this proved to be ideal for my mother who, at that time, was still alive but weak. With Dad away, she was relieved of her connection and could relax peacefully without interruption, stress, or worry.

6. INTERVIEWING AND HIRING HELP

Can you hire help? With the numbers of seniors increasing within Canada, more seniors' home-care service companies are opening. A qualified professional can tend to your parent's needs for a few hours and allow you some much-needed time and space.

If you have a nursing school in your city or town, you may be able to advertise for students to help. Attending students may be interested in picking up a part-time job for the extra income and to gain valuable related experience and a reference. When we were looking for someone to help with Dad, my family advertised in the local newspaper. This proved to be very effective. Place your ad in the weekend edition to take advantage of increased readership.

Probably the best way to find outside help is by referrals. Discuss with other caregivers what person or agency they would recommend. Choosing an independent respite provider will provide your parent with consistency (it will be the same face visiting); yet, a professional agency will have more staff available so you won't get caught unprepared. With coming from those in the similar situation as you are, you will be able to trust these recommendations.

Should you want to hire additional help, it is best to personally meet and interview applicants. By doing so, you will be able to gain a far better perspective on these individuals. While you are not permitted by law to probe applicants with personal questions (including details involving age, religious beliefs, place of birth, and political preferences), you are certainly entitled to ask for other facts. For interviewing purposes, try and meet somewhere comfortable for all parties and bring a list of questions so you do not forget anything. Design your questions to be more open-ended to encourage longer responses (simple "Yes" or "No" responses rarely tell you much about a person or his or her character). Here are a few ideas for questions you can ask:

- Tell me about yourself (the standard opening question for many interviews).
- Where have you worked before?
- What do you know about (name your own parent's health condition)?
- How do you handle stress and pressure? (You may want to ask the person to give an example to get a better understanding how he or she handles stress.)

- Why do you want this job?
- Tell me about a time when you had to adapt in a difficult situation.
- What skills have you acquired that you think would suit you for this job?

At the end of your interview, allow your applicant the opportunity to pose any questions in return. Not only is this common courtesy, it will demonstrate to you how enthusiastic this person is to work for you. With initial interviews, you are not required to talk salary, but you should come prepared with an idea of what pay range you are willing to offer. You also do not have to make any immediate hiring decisions. Take a few days to mull things over, debate applicants with other family members, and call the applicant's references. Personally, I encourage you to notify all potential applicants after you make a choice and courteously thank them for their interest.

Confirm that all workers are bonded, are physically able to lift and transfer your parent, and are trustworthy and dependable. Ask for two or three names as references, either personal or professional, and call these individuals.

You will want to observe how your new hire deals with your parent. This is perfectly understandable as he or she will be in a position of compassion, trust, and integrity.

Draft a short written agreement in which you can stipulate the hours of work and the rate of pay; have all parties involved sign this agreement. To avoid possible intimidation, title your agreement as something other than a "contract." You could refer to this as "terms of agreement" or "terms of hire" for example. Pay careful attention to outlining and itemizing the respite worker's exact responsibilities, such as whether you want him or her to entertain your parent with playing cards or something of the like. Or do you expect your respite worker to prepare dinner and do some additional housework? By fully spelling out responsibilities ahead of time, you can help to avoid uncertainty or assumptions. Have all parties sign and date the agreement, provide a copy to your new hire, and file one for yourself.

My family approached the care staff at Dad's facility to verify that our hired companion arrived as scheduled, until we found this no longer necessary to do. I also made several unscheduled visits to coincide with our worker's time there. I explained that my premise for visiting was for some other reason; however, my main purposes for stopping by were to ensure that she was onsite and to watch how she interacted with my father. I also designed a timesheet on which our caregiver noted her hours of work, plus explained any outings and activities, and noted any of Dad's behavioural changes. My family felt that writing this information down, helped to keep her accountable while also keeping us well informed.

If you are hiring outside help to come in for an afternoon or two per week, or to take your parent to an outside day program, help these other individuals get to know your parent. You can prepare a short list of your parent's likes and dislikes. Emphasize any irregular behaviours. Note regular medication times. Create a contingency plan so you will not be caught scrambling should plans change for the service provider.

7. MAKE SURE YOU SCHEDULE TIME FOR YOURSELF REGULARLY

No matter how you separate yourself from caregiving, book your own respite time regularly. Make a conscious effort to schedule time for just you. You will find at the end of this book a Scheduling "Me" Time form to help you manage your time. If the form doesn't work for you, use any other means that will work such as a reminder in your day planner, a comment on a wall calendar, or a note posted to your bathroom mirror. It is far better to maintain and moderate your personal health and well-being by looking out for yourself, rather than over-extend yourself and be of no service at all.

Assess your respite breaks. How much more relaxed did you feel afterward? You are looking for a positive self-report. Try different activities to figure out what most effectively relaxes you.

To stress my point about the importance of self-care, I would like to introduce you to two real individuals who took self-sacrifice to an extreme. First, a professional nurse who, frightening as it sounds, continually refused to drink water. This health-care worker's reasoning for reducing her water intake was that she would reduce her number of bathroom breaks, thus being able to spend more time with her patients. This same nurse also limited her lunch breaks and lingered after her shift longer than necessary because she found it difficult to allow someone else to take over. She changed her mind when she became pregnant — for her son to thrive, she had to thrive herself.

Next, a gentleman who, at a still young 45 years old, went to his doctor with complaints of light-headedness, nausea, dizziness, and shortness of breath. The diagnosis was that this man had suffered from a heart attack — not difficult to imagine because he was overweight. His extensive girth was caused by years of improper eating and lack of exercise — again, not putting himself first. Fortunately, the doctor caught this in time and this fellow decided to make dramatic lifestyle changes. Following open-heart surgery and becoming increasingly physically active, he reduced his weight and is far healthier and happier as a result.

While you will want to do everything possible to protect your loved one, you must also protect yourself. Do not compromise your own health and well-being. Despite a person's best intentions, caregiving can, and often does, become all-encompassing. By self-indulging a little rather than self-sacrificing, you will be a far better and more effective caregiver.

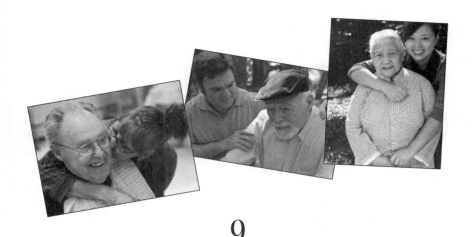

9
REMAINING ACTIVE

"Men must necessarily be the active agents of their own well-being and well-doing; they themselves must in the very nature of things be their own best helpers."

SAMUEL SMILES

Caregivers and loved ones should always take measures to remain active because this has been repeatedly proven to promote health. Physical activity will jump to mind for many. Remember, the body is a machine and it is meant to move, lift, twist, and turn. Keeping mobile also increases flexibility and circulation — just the thing for older bodies.

In my father's case, I recognized the need for physical activity and was strongly encouraged by facility care staff to take our regular walks. Walking with Dad had two benefits: it kept him mobile and provided an activity we could do together. Without these walks, Dad may have ended up in a wheelchair or, worse yet, a bucket chair, which is a demoralizing plastic scoop in which a person rests with both hands and feet off the floor. Like an overturned turtle, the person is unable to move. Another distressing option would have been for Dad to be physically restrained in a wheelchair. Granted, this happens for the individual's own safety because if he or she cannot stand, he or she cannot fall; however, where is the quality of life in that? Dad would never have understood being buckled in.

Thankfully, Dad's nursing home accommodated our walks. The family had appreciated the starfish-like design where each of the building's extended arms was another lengthy hallway. When the halls got jammed up with medical equipment or other residents or I got tired of the same scenery, I could always take Dad down to one of the lower floors. There was also a pleasant fenced-in back yard with a sidewalk; we could either loop around until Dad tired or just sit in the sun.

1. PREPARING AND TAKING YOUR PARENT FOR SEASONAL OUTINGS

If you can take your parent out but don't trust the weather, experiment with mall walking. Even in the most inclement weather, you can join others to stroll through a local shopping mall for socialization and exercise. If you can, find a mall-walking group in your city or town. If one does not exist, take the initiative and create your own. Talk to other family caregivers, post signage at the mall, and check with your local newspaper to ask if they will print your community announcement on an ongoing basis at no charge to you.

One word of caution though — heavy pedestrian traffic through a mall can be confusing and possibly dangerous for seniors. Drop in or call the shopping mall's administration office to ask when the mall is less busy. Sometimes, a shopping mall is opened earlier for the benefit of mall walkers. Senior visitors can quietly tour through while the stores are still closed. Granted, mall walkers will have to be earlier risers to take advantage of this arrangement, yet, without other shoppers constantly milling about, this can be very appealing.

If you do walk outside on a year-round basis, an elderly person will require some extra precautions. Aging skin becomes more sensitive to the sun. In the summertime, have your parent wear a broad-brimmed hat to protect him or her from sunburn. Long sleeves, even in warmer temperatures, will help to prevent sunburn and reduce insect bites. Don't forget to carry along plenty of mosquito repellent and extra sunblock.

In the wintertime, bundle up. Have your parent wear mittens, as these are warmer than gloves. On the fiercest Canadian winter days, wear a lighter pair of gloves underneath a pair of mittens — a simple but effective technique I call "double-gloving."

Look for a pair of winter boots for your parent that can easily slide on and off, offer stability, and which have a good tread for increased grip. A lower and flatter boot heel is also preferable and far more sensible. We found Dad a pair of winter boots with removable insoles, which could be slid out and dried easily.

A senior's winter jacket should extend past the waist to offer increased warmth and have conventional fasteners to keep things as simple as possible for both your hands and older hands that lack dexterity. Look for function over fashion! My father's parka, while warm enough, featured a double zipper. This proved to be more annoying than useful as the zipper would often refuse to slide up or down easily and get repeatedly caught in the fabric. It didn't take my sisters and I very long deciding to get a tailor to replace the zipper.

Your parent will remain much warmer when you dress him or her in layers. As with the winter parka, those additional layers should close with a zipper or buttons down the front of the garment. Crew neck sweaters, while fashionable, are challenging, if not impossible, for a senior to pull on. A material such as Thinsulate offers superb warmth without bulk or excessive weight.

When it comes to choosing your winter walking route, always stick with cleared sidewalks. Packed-down snow can look to be safe; however, it can be quite deceiving as it may hide treacherous black ice underneath. Excessive snow and ice build-up can be immensely risky for both of you to walk on. If you fall, your parent will likely tumble as well.

While you cannot totally prevent a fall, you can certainly limit the chances of this happening. One simple way to reduce the risk is with lightweight ice grips. Made of rubber and available in different sizes, these can be stretched over the sole of the shoe or boot to provide increased traction. With ice grips being quite popular with joggers and more serious runners, you will likely find these for purchase at your local sporting goods store.

If your loved one is in a wheelchair, stay clear of the snow as this makes pushing and navigating more difficult. You'll only have to try steering a wheelchair through deep snow once to agree.

Here are a few additional cold weather walking tricks so that "Old Man Winter" doesn't get the best of your parent:

- Pack along a small bag of cat litter. By sprinkling this on a slippery section of sidewalk, your parent can get a better grip and far safer footing.

- Walk slower and take smaller steps. When moving quickly across an icy surface, you are often asking for trouble. Depending on your parent's cognitive state, he or she may not even be aware that the snow and ice has become dangerous. As a caregiver, you must take the lead. By hesitating and keeping your feet closer together, you and your parent can achieve better balance and be able to stand and walk more securely.

- Experiment with a cane. A senior's cane can act as both an extra leg and an inquisitive finger. When using a cane, your parent can move more confidently on ice. A cane can also be used to reach out and poke at potentially threatening areas to ascertain how safe these areas will be. There are also cane ice grips, which are small teeth that can be attached to the end of a cane and raised or lowered as needed.

- Have your parent wear a belt. By grasping onto the belt (by the small of your parent's back) and holding on, you will be better able to steady him or her.

No matter what the season, when it comes to walking with your parent, you will have to remain extra attentive. Watch for cracks, uneven surfaces, and obstacles in your way. Even a branch on the sidewalk can pose a risk, because your parent may only shuffle rather than lift a foot to step over something.

Also, please walk with your loved one on the inside of the sidewalk, rather than on the outside. I am reminded of one day I took Dad out for a summer stroll. While I was tightly holding his arm to support him, Dad was walking on my left-hand side, next to the curb. I thought nothing of this but, in a moment of careless distraction, I loosened my grip on Dad's arm and he slipped and fell off the uneven curb. There are two important lessons here — always hold firmly and always be aware. Hitting the street, Dad cut his forehead open and started bleeding. While the cut was not serious, this caused me great angst; fortunately, a kind motorist stopped and offered us a ride back to the care facility where Dad was bandaged. Whether you are simply going around the block or straying further from the care facility, tuck your cell phone and a few extra dollars for cab fare into your pocket just in case.

2. FIND TIME FOR YOUR OWN PHYSICAL ACTIVITY

Find the time to keep physically active yourself. I liked to walk. This doesn't require any specialized sporting equipment. I didn't necessarily have to have any destination in mind. Sliding into a pair of comfortable shoes and getting outside often proved very therapeutic. The fresh air and movement was often helpful in reducing my stress level.

If you like more intense exercise, join a gym. To increase your workout regimen, choose a gym in your neighbourhood that you are comfortable with.

Gyms hold various advantages for members. You will frequently have others around to provide company and to spur you on. They will have qualified staff to teach you proper techniques. Also, your registration payment and ongoing membership dues can provide excellent inspiration for continuing to go.

If you cannot find the time to go to your gym three times per week, look at healthy alternatives, or "sneaky fitness" as I like to call it. Get creative with your ideas! Climb the stairs at your office building, park your car further away from the shopping mall door to encourage walking, take the dog for a walk, or do housework.

Try not to get caught up in the same routine either. Doing the same exercises will get boring quickly, and a boring exercise routine almost always gets dropped. Spice things up. In the spring or summer, you can go for a walk or run one day (alternate your routes and include a few hills to climb), play tennis the next, and go for a bicycle ride on another day. In the winter, don't let the colder temperatures hamper you; take up cross-country skiing or snow-shoeing, toboggan with your children, or swim at your neighbourhood pool. (Soak away some tension with a dip in the hot tub or a steam in the sauna afterward.) Enlist a friend to exercise with you to provide both companionship and motivation.

3. ACTIVITY ISN'T ALL ABOUT PHYSICAL EXERCISE

Exercise your mind as well. Don't ignore your brain's constant need to learn. Have you always wanted to study Japanese? Or learn how to make stained glass? What about a cooking course? Enroll in a class. This will stimulate your own brain and provide a welcome distraction from your caregiving duties. Classes, workshops, lectures, and seminars can also provide an excellent joint activity for you and your parent.

Read books on things you are interested in, not just information on your parent's medical condition and how to become a better caregiver. Pick up some books that are in your favourite genre. Frequent a second-hand bookstore as a means to experiment with new authors cost-effectively. Alternatively, support your local library with a membership. With this you will get almost unlimited book-borrowing privileges.

If you don't fancy yourself collecting even more books, consider purchasing an electronic reader where you can buy and store practically an unlimited supply of titles. These readers are both compact and slim enough to slide into a coat pocket, making them ideal for on-the-go caregivers; you will always have something new to read while waiting at the doctor's office.

With today's technology, you don't even need to curl up in your armchair to read. There are audiobooks that can be listened to in the car or while you are walking the dog. Local libraries often stock a wide selection of audiobooks to borrow.

Spiritual exercise is also important to maintain an overall individual balance. Practice and live your own faith, if applicable, as you would regularly do. Attend your church. Calm the racing thoughts through meditation or try a yoga class or Tai Chi.

As a caregiver, remain socially active and urge your parent to follow suit. If your parent remains lackadaisical about going out, arrange for neighbours to visit him or her. While we may not always crave companionship, human beings are social animals who enjoy spending time with others. Even a few words of conversation can make us feel better, more involved, and more mentally stimulated.

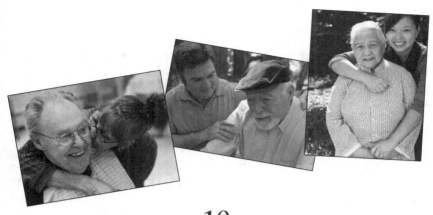

10
CAREGIVING VERSUS CAREER

Nothing is particularly hard if you divide it into small jobs.

HENRY FORD

As you will learn soon enough, or perhaps are learning right now, there are many roadblocks to being a caregiver. One of the most evident is that of one's own career. Employers may expect a minimum of 40 hours' work from you per week (more, if you work overtime). This can be both time-consuming and unrealistic when you are trying to balance additional caregiving responsibilities. Not to mention, a career can be mentally and physically tiring. Even if you can continually work these regular hours, you may come home at the end of the day exhausted with no energy to accomplish anything else. You will either push yourself closer to the brink (feeling a sense of obligation) or collapse on your couch. Either way, you are risking your own health and not doing your aged loved one, your family, or yourself any favours.

While there is no set time requirement for caregivers when it comes to providing eldercare, a realistic expectation would be that it will take at least 10 to 15 hours per week of personal time (this number can easily increase to 25 or 30 hours: almost a second full-time job). Where does this time come from? There are only 24 hours in each day. Unlike at work, caregivers don't function on a time clock. It's crucial to note that this caregiving time cannot always be precisely scheduled. An email request for a caregiver can arrive or a caregiver's phone can ring at any time with another task to do or, worse yet, an emergency situation. A person can do amazing things, at times, but working in excess of 70 hours per week (counting work plus caregiving) for any extended period of time can lead to breakdown or collapse.

I've experienced this problem previously. During my co-caregiving years, I recall trying desperately to find some kind of balance between my caregiving duties and my career. While I could — and did — ask for time off from my work in advance when I could, I did not always know when I would be needed. I've been remembering my father throughout this book for the most part, but a story about Mom seems to be most relevant now. With her leukemia, she required regular blood transfusions. These were lengthy sessions, with Mom remaining hooked up to an IV for hours. I had been called upon to drive her to the hospital one morning for this and had cleared it with my employer that I would arrive at work later than usual. As it turned out, Mom required some additional and unexpected medical testing and I remained to keep a watchful eye on the proceedings and to learn any news. This delayed my return to work and, when I did arrive at my desk, I was questioned and reprimanded by a very skeptical supervisor.

1. WORK OPTIONS

If an employer insists on your presence for a full work day, this may result in your squeezing in your caregiving tasks at other times and therefore making caregiving much less of a priority. I was stopping in to visit Mom and Dad on the way into work, slipping out at lunch to run a caregiving errand or two, or tending to a caregiving responsibility after leaving the job for the day. Perhaps you can relate?

It must be noted, however, that even when physically sitting at their desks, working caregivers may well be mentally distracted. Your mind may wander to thinking about a recent conversation you had with your parent's doctor, worrying, or running through a mental checklist of things you have to remember to do after work. Mental distractions such as these can easily lead to a lack of concentration on the job. When not completely focused, a caregiving employee can provide less than quality results, make mistakes, or even, depending on the job site, put him/herself (and others) at risk.

Another factor of concern for working caregivers is their own ability to sleep. If you have been lying awake since 3:00 a.m. the previous morning fretting or mentally reviewing tomorrow's schedule, you are going to be neither totally alert nor productive on the job the next day.

I like to think of myself as a fairly conscientious employee. I felt a strong sense of responsibility to fulfill my obligations, and therefore hesitated before taking a caregiving-related phone call while at work. You may feel guilty about doing so as well. Another issue for me was that I preferred to keep my personal matters to myself; a phone conversation at work could be easily overheard by someone in the next cubicle. And, if that phone call leads to your having to leave work suddenly, how do you explain it?

As a solution, it could be worthwhile to approach your employer and explain your current and anticipated situation before severe problems arise. With sufficient notice from you and some understanding and flexibility on your employer's part, a number of creative work options could be considered, such as:

- **Reducing your work hours:** Although this will affect your own monthly income, can you, even temporarily, lessen your time spent working? By doing so, you will be able to free up more of your own time to tend to your loved one's needs.

- **Working flex time:** Another option to consider is breaking up your work hours. Depending on the type of work that you do, it may well be possible to still get in eight hours per workday, but broken up so you can complete caregiving tasks in between work tasks. Perhaps you could rotate between a standard 9:00 a.m. to 5:00 p.m. shift one day and noon to 8:00 p.m. the next?

- **Taking a leave of absence:** Can you schedule some time away? Ideally, this would be paid time off, but there are no guarantees. With future health care for your loved one being uncertain (what, when, and how much will be needed), you cannot know how much leave to request. Realistically though, you will be asking for an extended leave of absence, but, of course, leaving that door open a crack to allow you the opportunity to return.

- **Working from home:** These days, with computers, cell phones, Skype, and email, people are always in touch. Can you set up a temporary home office (either in a second bedroom or on the dining room table) to serve as your workspace? If you can — and choose to — work from home, remember to provide some separation between your business and professional lives. I recall once telecommuting and using my home office for both work and as a storage area for a number of boxed files which I needed to refer to on a regular basis. With limited square footage and storage space in my home, there was little room for these boxes so, instead, I piled them in plain view in the middle of the floor. When I wrapped up my work day, I simply closed the door behind me so my work was not as conspicuous to my after-work life. If you are able to set yourself up to work at home, ensure that other people living in the same house respect your work space and time. You may have to insist on distraction-free time where you can concentrate on what needs to be done. If you are part of our country's sandwich generation and have young children yourself, this can make things even more difficult as toddlers aren't going to understand how to leave you alone (or even why this is necessary). In such cases, could your spouse mind the kids for a few hours, and, ideally, take them out of the house while you get some work done? Another idea would be to set up babysitting co-ops where neighbouring parents alternate monitoring young children at their homes so the other parents can better focus on work.

- **Job sharing:** In this situation, your job duties could be split and shared with another person. Your employer may like this plan if you offer to coach/mentor a new hire. Although there would be an additional salary to pay, it would be split with yours.

- **Temporary workers:** Can your employer approach a temporary work agency to contract short-term help in your absence? Temporary workers understand the nature of such employment and cannot have any expectations of a full-time, permanent offer. Therefore, when you are prepared to return to your job, the temporary worker can be easily released from duty.

Whatever terms you and your employer agree to should be written down. Don't count on a handshake deal or your own memory. Verbal agreements can be easily forgotten and human resource directors or your immediate supervisors can move on to other opportunities and be replaced. When this occurs, you will have to start negotiating again from square one making any previous discussion pointless. If nothing else, send a follow-up email summarizing your dialogue and understanding. By doing so, you will create a paper trail and have something to refer to if needed.

If things become too demanding, you may think about walking away from your employer completely. Granted, depending on your income level, your level of job satisfaction, and your seniority, this may be difficult. I well remember seriously considering giving my notice to leave my job, as I knew that my parents were my priority; while jobs can be replaced, parents cannot.

Think carefully before quitting in complete frustration and shutting the door on your employer. Ask yourself (or other family members or friends), "What am I leaving behind?" Work can provide mental stimulation, socialization, fulfillment, and a regular paycheck. Depending on how many years you have put in with a company, you may be provided with residual income in the form of a pension. If you leave on good terms, your employer will be more willing to invite you back, if and when the time arises, and/or provide you with a glowing reference letter praising your work should you decide to explore other potential jobs.

I'm a firm believer in not burning any bridges. No matter how difficult things may become, avoid leaving your employer on bad terms or without proper notice as this can scar your working reputation.

2. COMPASSIONATE CARE BENEFITS

For Canadian caregivers leaving their jobs, a financial safety net of sorts currently exists: Employment Insurance Compassionate Care Benefits. Workers who are supporting loved ones with serious health conditions can apply and receive up to 55 percent of their average insurable earnings. If you pursue this avenue, please note the following:

- benefits are presently limited to a maximum of six weeks,
- benefits are presently capped in the amount paid. Potential assistance will not exceed $485/week, and
- compassionate Care Benefits are taxable income.

For complete details and to see if you are eligible, please visit www.servicecanada.gc.ca/eng/ei/types/compassionate_care.shtml.

3. THINK BEFORE YOU LEAP

Resist jumping ship from your gainful employment too quickly. Remember that employees can be valuable commodities to employers. Considering your acquired job knowledge, stability, and valuable experience, your employer may not want to see you go. If your employer were to lose you, there could be an extensive hiring process required to replace you, including the cost of advertising, management time required to interview people, and training time for the new hire. These costs can work in your favour and be used as leverage.

There is also the trust factor. When you have been in your position for an extended period of time, your employer likely recognizes your ability to perform. With open discussion and as much notice as possible, you may be pleasantly surprised at the outcome. Your employer may come to you with an appropriate offer. Flexibility, for both parties, is the key here.

Findings from Health Canada's "National Profile of Family Caregivers in Canada — 2002: Final Report" (www.hc-sc.gc.ca/hcs-sss/pubs/home-domicile/2002-caregiv-interven/index-eng.php#a2_1) state, in part, that while many caregivers report difficulties balancing work and caregiving, 66 percent of those surveyed reported benefiting from flexibility from their employer. That same report continues to note that 42 percent of caregivers believe flexible work hours and provisions for short-term job and income protection from employers would be helpful.

I completely agree. Caregiving is not always to be expected by adult children, friends, partners, and spouses affected, and those providing care should not be penalized by losing out on regular income or a job because of circumstances beyond anybody's control. There has to be more compromising here. We don't normally ask to become caregivers and employers cannot, realistically, demand so much of a family caregiver's time and energy.

When it comes to finding an equitable balance between career and caregiving, there is no magic answer. Your situation, your priorities, and your life will be different from somebody else's. Such balance may easily change from one day to the next as well. As an example, my focus centred on me when I was single; however, now in a relationship, my attention has switched. You may have younger children who can easily place more demands on you from one day to the next. I cannot tell you that devoting a certain percentage of your time to one thing or another will or will not be appropriate as this is a personal choice. It should also be noted that, when I talk about a work-life balance, this does not necessarily mean an even split of your time and energy.

It's also important to try to not bring work home with you. While I could — and did — shut the second bedroom door to hide the stacked file boxes from view after working, I could not completely separate my two roles. If you have had a bad day at the office, do your best to leave those negative feelings at the office so your personal life and/or caregiving is not affected. A doctor I know came up with a simple answer to this problem; he would take 20 minutes just for himself on the drive home. He would go relax on a park bench or park in his own driveway to unwind before transitioning from busy doctor and health-care professional to husband and father.

As a final note here, I find it interesting but somewhat disappointing that many employers will support their staff with personal issues including providing maternity leave, addictions counselling, and paid training programs, but continue to turn a blind eye toward the needs of those involved with eldercare.

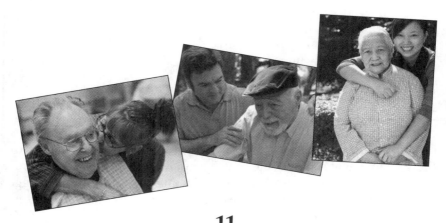

11
MOBILITY AIDS AND EMERGENCY SAFETY DEVICES FOR SENIORS

"Remember, if you ever need a helping hand, it's at the end of your arm. As you get older, remember you have another hand: The first is to help yourself, the second is to help others."

AUDREY HEPBURN

This chapter will introduce you to a number of helpful mobility aids to make a senior's life easier. It's important to purchase these items from reputable, established dealers and ensure there is a warranty or exchange program in place. With personal items, carefully consider the fit. Can your parent be sized or is the item adjustable? Of course, there are many mobility aids and other products on the market, with more being developed each day. Here is a small sampling of large and small products that can dramatically help your parents in their daily lives.

You will also find information in this chapter about safety devices that can help protect your loved one.

1. MOBILITY AIDS AND OTHER USEFUL ITEMS

Browse through your local daily living store for seniors' aids and you may be amazed at what you can find. If you don't spot something on the shelves, mention this to store staff. They may be able to special-order something in for you or serve as a direct pipeline to the manufacturers to invent a new product.

1.1 Walk-in bathtubs

These ingenious tubs make bathing easier and safer for a senior. A door or sliding panel in the side of the tub can be opened by someone prior to taking a bath. Water pressure ensures a tight seal, so there is no leakage. The senior can easily step in, rather than up and over the bathtub edge, and sit down. Thanks to walk-in tubs, aging parents can bathe without worries and therefore are able to remain independent for a longer period of time.

1.2 Stair lifts

A common set of stairs can become a huge obstacle for someone without the strength to climb them. The second floor of a home can become completely shut off because a senior may not be able to gain access.

As I witnessed with my mother, stairs into the home can be restrictive. Consider that the entrance stairs may pose a risk; for example, not only could a senior trip and face potential injury, he or she could be trapped inside the home and unable to escape in the case of a fire or other emergency.

With a powered stair lift, your parent can smoothly ride up and down a staircase using a hand-held remote. Look for a stair lift with battery backup. Should there be a power outage, you will not want your parent to be stranded halfway between floors.

1.3 Lift chairs

Combining comfort and convenience, lift chairs make it easier for an individual to sit or stand. Your parent can simply back up into the chair and be gradually lowered to a sitting position. Standing from the chair is equally easy as the user can press a button to have the chair gradually rise and tilt forward. (Note that sizing is important here — one size does not fit everybody.) When a person is sitting properly, his or her knees should be bent at right angles with feet flat on the floor.

Lift chairs are available in an array of colours and models with various reclining positions for the increased comfort of the user.

Your parent can sit upright, lean back to watch television, or recline fully for an afternoon nap.

1.4 Walkers

If your mother or father is not restricted to a wheelchair or bed, a walker can help with more secure standing and moving around. A walker must be sized correctly for the individual using it (Mom or Dad will have to lean forward slightly to hold on, but should remain upright when using a walker) and it will feature a hand brake to stop this mobility aid from dangerously rolling forward or backward without notice.

Many walkers can also be transformed into chairs, which is perfect for the tiring senior to use for resting. There are also a variety of colourful and useful bags that can be attached to a walker for handy storage.

1.5 Scooters

Scooters are mechanical devices that provide increased mobility along with safety. Mobility scooters are usually powered by a rechargeable battery system and come with various options.

Before purchasing a scooter, carefully consider the intended usage. Key questions to ask include:

- Where will the scooter be used?
- For what purpose will the scooter be used?
- Will the scooter be easily transportable?
- Can the scooter be easily disassembled?

A three-wheeled model will be quite nimble and perfect for tight maneuvering inside of a home, while a four-wheeled model is built for the outdoors and will be far more stable and rugged. Convincing your parent to take a scooter for a test drive may take some time as the transition to a scooter may be viewed as unnecessary. However, once your parent is in the driver's seat and enjoying enhanced independence, he or she may quickly change in mindset. With both walkers and scooters, take time to disassemble and reassemble them at the store prior to purchase. Don't just watch the salesperson do this; he or she can demonstrate a product repeatedly and the process will appear to be smooth and easy.

1.6 Grab bars

Install grab bars firmly along walls, ensuring they are well within reach. Such grab bars can be placed throughout a senior's home; however, they are used most frequently in the bathroom. Grab bars can help a senior sit down and stand up from the toilet, pull himself or herself out of the bathtub, or steady himself or herself in the shower.

1.7 Grab poles

My sisters and I found an adjustable pole that could be braced between the floor and the ceiling beside a bed. This was more for Mom's sake. As she was quite weak, the pole was useful to help her pull herself out of bed.

1.8 Reachers

Reachers are an excellent invention implementing a hand-held pole with a set of moving pinchers on one end. These pinchers can be opened and closed, allowing the senior to grasp something off a higher shelf or just out of reach on the floor.

1.9 Faucet grippers

These enlarged plastic covers slide over existing taps so they can be turned on and off with ease, even with arthritic joints. I found a set that featured bright red and blue grippers to allow for quick differentiation between water temperatures. Even if someone had limited visibility, these vibrant colours could be seen.

1.10 Magnifying glass

Older eyes will have more difficulty reading smaller print. When shopping for a magnifying glass, choose one with a wider or heavier handle, making it easier to grasp.

There are also illuminated magnifying sheets, which are large enough to place over a book page.

1.11 Large-buttoned telephone

Large-buttoned telephones may look odd, but they can be of tremendous value to seniors. The oversized buttons are not only easier to see, they are also much easier to press.

1.12 Bell

In this case a bell is not for home decoration. A bell can be a very useful item for a senior still living at home. In times of distress, the bell can be rung and the sound can, typically, be heard throughout a home. You can place bells in various locations throughout the home. I highly recommend putting a bell in the bathroom. You will often see emergency call buttons or pull cords in hospital bathrooms — these are installed for very good reasons.

1.13 Non-slip grip mat

A non-slip grip mat can be of tremendous value in the bathroom. Wet floors can prove to be highly slippery and an unsteady senior could easily fall.

1.14 Wall calendar

Hang a wall calendar in a conspicuous area where your parent can see it. I like the monthly calendar format rather than a dayplanner because it can better show scheduled appointments ahead of time. Choose a wall calendar with large enough squares should you need to write in multiple appointments on one day. You might even try colour-coding scheduled appointments. Write down the important doctor's appointment in red ink, the weekly visit to church in blue ink, and other intermittent events in black ink. Use darker ink so it's easier to read.

1.15 Raised toilet seats

These can become handy for seniors who may encounter difficulties going to the bathroom. Such seats can be either connected to the toilet base or be portable for easier storage and travelling. With a brace bolted to the floor or a grab bar installed on the wall beside the toilet, your parent will always have a helping hand, even if you are not there to help.

1.16 Weighted cutlery

While you and I may not think twice about picking up a fork to eat our meals, seniors can fight with this seemingly simple task. Eating can become frustrating, if not impossible, if a senior's hands continually shake from arthritic tremors. With unsteady hands, food can continually fall from the fork or spoon. The senior can more confidently hold and use heavier cutlery, thus providing him or her an increased sense of pride because he or she can continue to feed himself or herself and not rely on caregiver assistance.

There is also a wide range of ergonomically designed forks, spoons, and knives on the market to make for easier feeding. These specially designed utensils are also good for a senior that has use of only one hand.

1.17 Medication reminder

A medication reminder is very simple, yet highly effective, product. You can often find these at your local drugstore. A medication reminder is often a plastic box with individual compartments marked for each day of the week or separated into day parts (i.e., morning and evening, or breakfast, lunch, and dinner).

If you are picking up prescriptions for your parent from the pharmacy, you can also provide the medication blister packs to institution staff to split up as needed. Caregivers can separate different prescription medication and place pills in each compartment. Doing this will provide an excellent visual for your parent to take the pills. This will also be useful for any visiting caregiver if he or she will be with your mother or father at medication time. The caregiver can simply be directed to give that specific day's pills. Finally, a medication reminder will help you, the caregiver, to see if your parent did take the prescribed pills.

1.18 Pill crusher

Depending on your parent's health needs, a handful of medications may be prescribed. That handful of pills, both in quantity and in potential size, may be difficult to take. With a pill crusher, medication can be split or ground down into easier-to-ingest powder. If your parent hesitates to take prescribed medication, grind the pills down and mix them in ice cream or pudding.

1.19 Cushions

Cushions come in many shapes and sizes and also vary immensely in firmness. You can place a cushion on a chair for increased comfort, use one when sleeping, or slide one into one side of a wheelchair to help prop up your parent, should your parent have posture problems. Check what kind of filling the cushion has if your parent has allergies to any type of materials.

2. EMERGENCY SAFETY DEVICES

Numerous safety and security products are also available for seniors — some examples of these products are explained in the following sections. With any alarm system, be cognizant of how the alert is sounded; for example, a flashing light corresponding to a room number may be temporarily overlooked by a nurse distracted by another resident. Therefore, it is recommended to look at both auditory and visual alarms.

2.1 Personal security alarms

Typically worn around the neck as a pendant, personal security alarms are commonly patched directly through to an around-the-clock call centre. Watchful staff can immediately notify you, call the neighbours, or dispatch an ambulance to the senior's residence.

2.2 MedicAlert bracelets

Far more than just attractive jewellery, MedicAlert bracelets can be engraved with a senior's personal health records, allergies, or current diagnosis. Should a senior require immediate care, proper help can be provided without lengthy delays. You will want to ensure a MedicAlert bracelet fits well around your parent's wrist and that it will not irritate his or her skin.

2.3 Emergency telephone call buttons

Emergency telephone call buttons are often programmed to reach the facility's front office or nursing station. With a single push of the button, an alert will be sounded and help can arrive quickly. While the one-button operation provides ease of use for a senior in need, the telephone must be within easy reach for the button to be most effective.

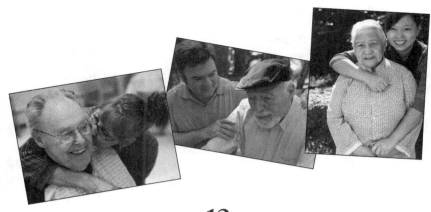

12
FINDING JOY IN CAREGIVING

"What seems to us as bitter trials are often blessings in disguise."

OSCAR WILDE

Caring for both my mother and father were some of the hardest things I have ever had to do; I was neither expecting nor prepared for this role. Watching a parent decline without being able to help can be a very complicated matter. Personally, I helplessly witnessed many changes in my father; certainly one of the most apparent was the complete loss of his mental faculties. Dad, once an avid book-lover, was reduced to being barely able to grasp a book in his hands, and with only the faintest recognition.

You too can expect a difficult journey. Caregiving can be try-ing because you can be torn physically, mentally, and emotionally in many different directions, simultaneously. You may be stretched to your very limits and then even past these limits. As a caregiver, you may find there are not enough hours in the day or days in a week to accomplish everything that needs to be done. As a caregiver, you may be run ragged trying to balance everything, but you will need to endure.

Surprisingly, caregiving can also be a beautiful thing. This may seem contradictory to you, yet during these most difficult times, you can develop and forge stronger family relationships, open lines of communication between parents and siblings, become better organized, and strengthen your own personal resolve. Like a needle in a haystack, those joyous times in caregiving may be difficult to find. When preoccupied with tending to your parent's immediate needs, you may not even recognize the good times until years later — perhaps even after your parent is gone. You can consider these hidden gems that you will fondly hold close.

I do not believe that caregiving is either burdensome or obligatory. You are simply returning the favour to your parents who tended to your needs as a growing child. You might feel it is now your turn. When approaching this role properly, you will find your own inner strengths and survive because doing this will make you a stronger, more confident, mature, compassionate, better, and wiser person. Whether it is through the touch of your parent's hand, a soft kiss, a smile, another expression of love, or a confession made, you may find moments which move you or draw you much closer to your mother or father. While I lost my father twice (once when he forgot who I was and again when he passed away), I also gained a father I never truly knew. While you may have heard of many horror stories relating to caregiving and senior care, know that this is *not* all doom and gloom.

To further explain, my father was always an intensely private man. I never really knew him. I only grasped this in his later years when I finally began to understand his nature. As a result of Alzheimer's disease, Dad was unable to hide behind his emotionally protective wall any longer and his true personality and characteristics emerged. I could better see who Dad was as his wall crumbled. The cards that he had been dealt in life became more apparent. As an only child, Dad looked to his parents for love and support. My grandfather died when Dad was quite young, leaving only him as a small boy, and his mother.

Without that father figure of his own, Dad had no role model to follow. I am not a parent myself but recognize that much of parenthood is learning as one goes, which is very similar to caregiving. Mirroring one's own experience can be very helpful. Dad had no such experience but was the best father he could be, given what he had. With Alzheimer's disease, this aging man became a fun-loving child — a child with a kind, gentle soul who liked to be hugged. Although Dad could not remember, he remained a human being, deserving of the utmost respect, care, quality of life, and dignity.

With joy comes laughter. Although caregiving is a serious matter, allow yourself to laugh. While I have been remembering Dad throughout this book, I well recall a moment with my mother. During a visit with her, Mom slipped and fell on the floor. Concerned, I immediately rushed to her, and, much to my surprise, she started laughing! Mom always had a quirky sense of humour. Thankfully, she was absolutely fine. Her reason for laughing, she explained, was that she felt like an overturned turtle, too weak to right herself or stand up again. To emphasize that point, she ineffectively weakly waved her arms and legs in the air. Greatly relieved, I laughed with her, extended my hand and then helped her to her feet. As a caregiver, you will have tremendous responsibility on your shoulders, but this does not mean that you must be serious all the time.

There are many other joys involved with caregiving. You will increase your opportunities for self-discovery. Although your learning curve may be steep, you will learn about your parent's condition as well as your own abilities. Always remember, you can succeed.

You will discover who your true friends are. These friends will be the ones who will continually support, encourage, and listen to you without judgment. These friends will not only offer to help you in whatever way they can, they will follow through on commitments.

You will become better organized. There is nothing like minding your parent's matters to teach you improved organizational skills. If you have not done so already, caregiving can also remind you to get your own affairs in order. Have you drafted up your own will?

You will be far happier if you remain easy on yourself. Your body will tell you when you are doing too much. It is up to you to listen to and acknowledge those messages. You are only one person and, for this reason alone, it is imperative for you to seek out caregiving help and to take your own personal respite time. It is not my intention to preach but only to advise and guide you as you look ahead. Knowing everything that lies ahead for you as a caregiver is impossible, but you can begin to prepare yourself.

One of the best things that you can do for yourself and your loved one is to accept. Accept your own limitations. Accept what you cannot change. Everybody makes mistakes. We humans are not perfect, nor can we ever be perfect. Recognize your own human restrictions.

Accept time limitations. There are only 24 hours in a day. With 8 hours required for a good night's sleep and 8 hours on the job, two-thirds of your days are spoken for. In the remaining time, you must juggle other responsibilities including your own family, housework, and shopping. Don't short-change yourself on sleep to give yourself more time during the day.

Accept the cards you have been dealt in life. While you may feel you have been given a terrible hand, these same cards can offer many other rewards — both large and small.

Congratulate yourself often for what you do. Not everybody can, or will, become a caregiver. You have chosen this path and committed to see it through to the end. Not everybody has the fortitude to do this and you are to be admired.

While I have tried to provide directions and advice to you, I certainly do not have all the answers. A guidebook such as this can only provide a general idea of how to deal with your situation. There is no complete caregiving road map or any directional road signs, because each tool would be inadequate — every caregiver's starting points and destinations vary. Each caregiver can be vastly different as well. With that said, you will find similarities between caregivers' personal stories, which include both tragedies and triumphs.

Good luck and best wishes on your own caregiving journey. Make yourself and your parents proud!

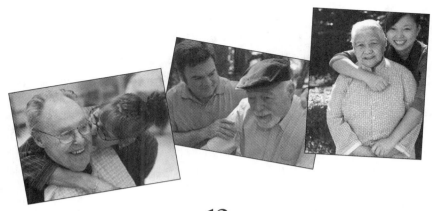

13
FINAL THOUGHTS

"Final thoughts are so, you know, final. Let's call them closing words."

CRAIG ARMSTRONG

While this book is now coming to a close, know that your own caregiving story is just beginning. Your parent will develop as the lead character and you will serve in a supporting role. Your own storyline will unfold as you fulfill your various caregiving responsibilities. There are an unknown number of chapters ahead of you; however, you will learn, manage, grow stronger, and experience both joy and sorrow.

If you find yourself questioning yourself as a caregiver, know this is to be expected — being human, you can only do so much. When you feel self-doubt creeping in or lingering with you, glance through the following words of advice. I have listed these in bullet form to provide you a quick and easy read.

- Take time for yourself regularly. I've prioritized this as the first point because it is the most important but most often overlooked point for caregivers.
- Know that you are never alone as a caregiver.
- Prepare for the future.
- Remain flexible with your time.
- Enlist the help of family, friends, and health-care workers.

- Allow others to help you when they offer.
- Think outside of the box. Who else can help you and how?
- Accept your own, and others', limitations.
- Set achievable caregiving goals.
- Share your caregiving heartaches and successes with those you love.
- Trust your instincts.
- Allow yourself to cry, if need be.
- Take time for yourself regularly. (Yes, I have mentioned this before, but it bears repeating.)
- Remember that there is joy in caregiving even though it may not be immediately obvious.
- Continue to learn everything you can about your parent's health condition.
- Treat your parent with respect and dignity. Your parent remains a human being.
- Ensure that your parent is enjoying the best quality of life possible.
- Keep your parent comfortable.
- Love your parent unconditionally.
- Manage your parent's affairs ethically.
- Protect your parent from possible physical, mental, emotional, and financial abuse.
- Take pride in what you do as a caregiver.
- Work to release yourself of any lingering self-doubt and guilt that you are not doing enough as a caregiver.
- Value your time and efforts as a caregiver.
- Exercise patience with yourself, your parent, and others.
- Maintain open lines of communication between all parties involved. Share and listen.
- Decide what you can do and what you cannot do as a caregiver.
- Understand that grieving a loss can begin even before death.

- Seek out caregiving coping mechanisms that can work for you.
- Reflect on what is most important in your life and your parent's life.
- Ask yourself, "What would Mom or Dad do or want in this situation?"
- Strive for balance in your own personal and professional lives.
- Expect and embrace uncertainty with how to proceed with caregiving.
- Communicate with your own family.
- Dismiss self-doubt that you cannot provide adequate or quality care for your parent.
- Avoid sacrificing your own life for another's.
- Rest when needed.
- Explain your impending need for time away from work with your employer ahead of time. Discuss possible work arrangements including paid leave, reduced hours, or work-sharing with another individual.
- Lobby politicians for increased caregiver funding, tax breaks, and service or support programs at civic, provincial, and national levels.
- Again: take time for yourself regularly. Please do not forget your own needs.

RESOURCES

As a caregiver, you are reaching out to people, but when you need help, where will you turn? I have researched a number of Canadian-specific senior- and caregiving-related websites and I am pleased to share these with you here. Find the websites of most use or relevance to you, then "bookmark" them so you can easily find them again later.

1. ORGANIZATIONS, ASSOCIATIONS, AND GOVERNMENT AGENCIES

Advocacy Centre for the Elderly

A Toronto community-based legal clinic for low-income seniors and the first Canadian legal clinic specializing in seniors' legal issues.

www.advocacycentreelderly.org

Alberta Seniors and Community Supports

This site includes a link to the Alberta *Supportive Living Accommodation Licensing Act,* which was implemented in April 2010. Through this legislation, family caregivers can better ensure that facilities are properly equipped and licensed to provide the highest quality of care. Inquiring family caregivers either living in Alberta (or moving their parent to this province) can now window shop the seniors' accommodation available to them. If you do not have similar legislation in your province, push your local politicians to take action in this direction.

You can investigate all licensed senior facilities in Alberta, compare accommodation details, check out the number of registered complaints and even learn the eligibility for supplied government funding. This website is a tremendous resource for those who can take advantage of it.

http://asalreporting.gov.ab.ca/astral

Canada Mortgage and Housing Corporation

Home Adaptations for Seniors' Independence (HASI)

Offering a financial-assistance program for low-income seniors requiring minor home adaptations.

www.cmhc-schl.gc.ca/en/co/prfinas/prfinas_004.cfm

Canada Safety Council

Home Adaptation Checklist

Including a helpful and complete home adaptation checklist of what you can do to make your parent's home a safer place.

https://Canadasafetycouncil.org/home-safety/home-adaptation-checklist

Canadian Association of Retired Persons (CARP)

A society advocating for quality of life, financial, and health security, as well as human rights for aging Canadian seniors.

www.carp.ca

Canadian Caregiver Coalition (CCC)

This office advocates for Canadian caregivers, develops social innovation, and schedules special events.

www.ccc-ccan.ca

Canadian Home Care Association (CHCA)

The national voice of home care in our country. CHCA ensures the accessible delivery of appropriate heath-care services to seniors living at home.

www.cdnhomecare.ca

Canadian Hospice Palliative Care Association

This office advances and advocates for quality end-of-life hospice palliative care.

www.chpca.net/home.html

Canadian National Institute for the Blind (CNIB)

The CNIB provides information, support, and hope to our country's visually impaired.

www.cnib.ca

Citizenship and Immigration Canada

Canadian Work Permits

This is an application for workers from outside of Canada who wish to work in our country on a temporary basis.

www.cic.gc.ca/english/information/applications/work.asp

The Live-in Caregiver Program

Providing a comprehensive listing of requirements for those wishing to work as live-in caregivers.

www.ci.gc.ca/english/work/caregiver/apply-who.asp

Government of Canada (and Seniors Canada)

Healthy Canadians

Including must-know information on food warnings, advisories, and recalls.

www.healthycanadians.gc.ca/index-eng.php

National Seniors Council

Advises on current and emerging senior-related issues in our country.

www.seniorscouncil.gc.ca/eng/home.shtml

Elder Abuse

This link takes you to the Seniors Canada homepage.

www.seniors.gc.ca/eng/index.html

The following link takes you to information on elder abuse.

www.seniors.gc.ca/eng/sb/ie/index.html

Veterans Affairs Canada

This site is provided by the Government of Canada and gives you information about veterans' affairs such as pension, benefits, and financial sources.

www.veterans.gc.ca

Health Canada

This site provides the story behind the news on food recalls and warnings. It also includes valuable information on drugs and health products, consumer product safety, and Canada's health system.

www.hc-sc.gc.ca

You can order your free copy of *Eating Well with Canada's Food Guide* online or by calling 1-800-926-9105.

www.hc-sc.gc.ca/fn-an/food-guide-aliment/index-eng.php

Human Resources and Skills Development Canada

Canadian Pension Plan and Old Age Security

A comprehensive overview of these financial benefit plans for Canada's seniors.

Learn more about Canada's retirement income system and review required documents for application.

www.hrsdc.gc.ca/eng/oas-cpp/index.shtml

Hiring a Live-In Caregiver

This site outlines the application process for those wishing to work as a live-in caregiver; it also explains the foreign live-in caregiver program and lists the obligations of employers.

www.hrsdc.gc.ca/eng/jobs/foreign_workers/caregiver/index.shtml

International Federation on Ageing (IFA)

This site is a point of connection, information sharing and exchange, research, and advocacy and policy knowledge for seniors.

www.ifa-fiv.org

Public Health Agency of Canada

Working to prevent and control infectious and chronic diseases. Promoting good health for seniors.

www.phac-aspc.gc.ca/index-eng.php

Publications of the Division of Aging and Seniors

A complete alphabetical list of available resources is included on this site. Publications can either be read online or ordered.

www.phac-aspc.gc.ca/seniors-aines/publications/index-eng.php

Public Trustees, Guardians, and Administrators

The following link takes you to the Government of Alberta site. It gives you links to public trustees, guardians, and administrators for all the provinces and territories.

humanservices.alberta.ca/guardianship-trusteeship/opg-other-provinces.html

Canada Revenue Agency (CRA)

Claiming the Caregiver Amount

Do you know what the CRA caregiver amount is and how you can claim it? This site will help you find the answers.

www.cra-arc.gc.ca/tx/ndvdls/tpcs/ncm-tx/rtrn/cmpltng/ddctns/lns300-350/315

Service Canada

Guaranteed Income Supplement (GIS)

Offering a definition of the GIS and a review of the application process.

www.servicecanada.gc.ca/eng/isp/pub/oas/gismain.shtml

Income Security Programs

A point of contact for seniors and caregivers with questions regarding income Old Age Security and Canada Pension Plan programs.

www.servicecanada.gc.ca/eng/isp/contact/contact_us.shtml

Forms of Assistance for Caregivers

What caregivers will need to get started with applying for employment insurance, compassionate care benefits, and claiming the caregiver amount on a tax return.

www.servicecanada.gc.ca/eng/lifeevents/caregiver.shtml

Telecare Distress Centres of Canada

Lonely? Frustrated? Stressed? This office provides somewhere to call and someone to listen. This service is available across Canada.

www.telecarecanada.org

Veterans Affairs Canada

Provides information about veterans' services and benefits, applying for a pension, and obtaining military service records.

www.veterans.gc.ca

Caregivers' Rights

This link includes a handy list about caregivers' rights. Print off a copy and place it in a prominent place.

www.veterans.gc.ca/eng/health/caregiving

Veterans Independence Program (VIP)

Provides complete details on the Veterans Independence Program, which is a national home-care program provided by Veterans Affairs Canada.

www.veterans.gc.ca/eng/services/veterans-independence-program/apply

Provincial Caregiver Associations

While the Canadian Caregivers Association acts as an umbrella organization and serves all of our country's caregivers, some provinces and territories have localized offices. One of the following offices may be more convenient for you to reach.

Family Caregivers' Network Society — British Columbia
www.fcns-caregiving.org

Alberta Caregivers Association
www.albertacaregiversassociation.org

Caregiver Information and Support — Saskatchewan
www.saskatooncaregiver.ca/index.html

Victorian Order of Nurses — Manitoba
www.von.ca/en/NationalDirectory/branch.aspx?BranchId=15

Caring for a Senior — Ontario
www.ottawa.ca/residents/public-health/healthy-living/caring-senior

Association des Aides Familiales du Quebec
www.aafq.ca

Caregivers Nova Scotia
www.caregiversns.org

Hospice Palliative Care Association of Prince Edward Island
www.hospicepei.ca

Seniors Resource Centre of Newfoundland & Labrador
www.seniorsresource.ca/caregivers/index.htm

2. OTHER USEFUL LINKS

The Care Guide
This site includes everything under the sun for seniors' housing and care.
www.thecareguide.com/home.aspx

Complete Canadian Wills Kit and Power of Attorney Kit
Save legal costs by writing your own will and power of attorney.
www.self-counsel.com

Hospice Net
While this is an American website, Canadian caregivers may still learn valuable information regarding hospices and hospice care.
www.hospicenet.org

Mama's Health
This site includes information on how to choose a doctor for a senior as well as topics on Alzheimer's disease, hip fractures, long-term care, (and more).
www.mamashealth.com/senior/doctor.asp

MedicAlert Canada
This site will provide you with all you need to know about MedicAlert.
www.medicalert.ca

Philips Lifeline Canada
A personal response service to summon help if needed.
www.lifeline.ca

3. ARTICLES ON THE INTERNET

The Internet is one of the best resources for caregivers. When you feel like you may have nowhere to turn and there is no one to answer your questions, try typing a few words relating to what you are looking for into a search engine. By doing so, you can quickly and simply find information on practically any topic you want to know more about. You may want to confirm the information you find online has been provided by a trustworthy source. The following articles are just a few preliminary examples and may well be relevant to you (either now or in the future).

Cleaning Your Wheelchair Cushion to Extend Its Life
http://www.spinlife.com/spintips/details/k/Clean%20Your%20
Wheelchair%20Cushion%20to%20Extend%20its%20Life/a/118/c/89

Depression in Caregivers
http://alzheimers.about.com/cs/frustration/a/depression.htm

How to Care for Eyeglasses
www.ehow.com/how_2050918_care-eyeglasses.html

How to Care for Hearing Aids
http://www.ehow.com/how_2057343_care-hearing-aids.html

How to Care for Your Dentures
http://dentistry.about.com/od/falseteeth/a/carefordentures.htm

How to Size a Walking Cane
www.ehow.com/how_5600909_size-walking-cane.html

Manual Wheelchair Maintenance
http://www.spinlife.com/spintips/details/k/Manual%20Wheelchair
%20Maintenance/a/116/c/2

Mobility Scooters Buyer's Guide and FAQ
www.wheelchairguide.net/mobility-scooter-buyers-guide-faq

Senior Driving
www.helpguide.org/elder/senior_citizen_driving.htm

Your Annual Checkup
http://seniorhealth.about.com/cs/prevention/a/checkup.htm

CAREGIVING CHECKLISTS
AND WORKSHEETS

1. YOUR CIRCLE OF CAREGIVING

As a caregiver, you can surround yourself with outside resources. Take some time to identify family, friends, colleagues, associations, seniors' programs, and services that can help you. It's not necessary to complete this assignment in one sitting; you will add more names to your circle as you proceed. Please also enlarge this circle as required. These will be new people you meet or organizations of which you will learn. Having more helping hands involved with your parent's care will, ultimately, help you as a caregiver.

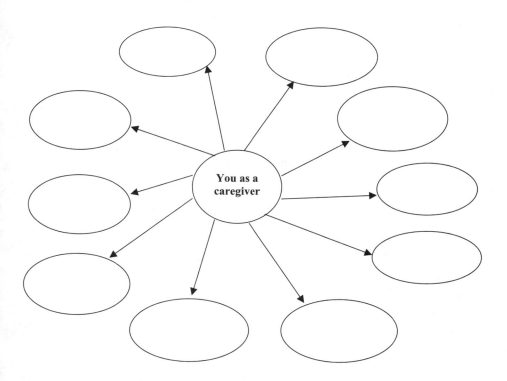

2. SCHEDULING "ME" TIME

Don't ever ignore the need for personal respite! As a caregiver, you will need to remove yourself regularly from the situation to prevent things from becoming too overwhelming. Looking after your own self-interests is not being self-centered; doing this is being self-protective. Make photocopies of this page and use it to schedule some personal time for you. Keep to this schedule as best you can. Monitor your results; you will feel better and more in control.

Activity: _____

Day: _____

Time of day and time required: _____

Personal rewards: _____

Activity: _____

Day: _____

Time of day and time required: _____

Personal rewards: _____

Activity: _____

Day: _____

Time of day and time required: _____

Personal rewards: _____

Activity: _____

Day: _____

Time of day and time required: _____

Personal rewards: _____

Activity: _____

Day: _____

Time of day and time required: _____

Personal rewards: _____

Activity: _____

Day: _____

Time of day and time required: _____

Personal rewards: _____

Activity: _____

Day: _____

Time of day and time required: _____

Personal rewards: _____

Activity: _____

Day: _____

Time of day and time required: _____

Personal rewards: _____

3. CAREGIVING SELF-ANALYSIS

Self-evaluation is crucial to caregivers. While you will be presented with many new challenges, you must know what you can do and the extent of your own limits. Answer the following questions as honestly as you can. Addressing these issues sooner, rather than later, will help you identify your own strengths and weaknesses and will be beneficial to you as a caregiver. Share these questions with your siblings and delegate your roles appropriately.

1. What can you do as a caregiver?
2. How do you feel about becoming and acting as a caregiver?
3. What would you identify as your characteristic strengths and weaknesses?
4. Who will help you with your caregiving responsibilities?
5. How will others help you with your caregiving duties? (Identify what others can do.)
6. Beyond your immediate circle of contacts, where will you look for additional help?
7. Can you work easily with others or do you like to work independently?
8. Are you flexible with your own schedule?
9. What negative issues do you foresee with serving as a caregiver?
10. How will you respond to or counteract these negative issues?
11. Where will you seek respite for your loved one?
12. Where will you seek respite for yourself?
13. List three additional ideas for personal coping and caring mechanisms (these will be new areas of interest to you that you could try in the future).
14. How much personal respite time will you give yourself?
15. What do you want to achieve as a caregiver?
16. Are you hesitant or reluctant to serve as a caregiver? If so, why?
17. How much will this hesitation interfere with your caregiving duties? Will you be able to perform certain tasks or do you need to assign them to others?

18. Can you honestly look at yourself in the bathroom mirror and say, "I am doing the best job I can as a caregiver"?

19. Do you have any regrets about serving as a caregiver? If so, what are your regrets and how can you resolve them?

20. Where can you learn more about your loved one's medical condition and prognosis?

21. What other personal and professional demands, besides caregiving, exist for you?

22. How will you know you have done your best being a caregiver?

23. Are you an optimist or a pessimist? (Note that optimists will have an easier time and might be better caregivers.)

4. CAREGIVER'S DOCUMENT WORKSHEET

Complete the following worksheet to keep vital personal information handy. Use a separate sheet for further information, if necessary. Provide photocopies of this list to your other siblings. Store your own copy in a secure place such as your home safe.

Personal Records:

Parent's complete name: _____

Maiden name: _____

Nickname(s): _____

Social Insurance Number: _____

Birth date: _____

Birth place: _____

Age: _____

Citizenship status: _____

Military service: _____

Bank(s): _____

Bank branch address: _____

Bank branch phone number: _____

Bank account number(s): _____

Financial holdings (e.g., mutual funds): _____

Investments: _____

Sources of income (e.g., pension, savings): _____

Amount of regular pension cheques: _____

(Find the following information and obtain originals of these documents or, at least, know where to find them.)

Driver's licence number: _____

Birth certificate: _____

Marriage licence(s): _____

Divorce record(s): _____

Property titles (both real estate and land): _____

Insurance policies (e.g., life, homeowner's, health): _____

Tax Records: _____

Will: _____

Advance directive: _____

Credit cards: _____

Personal property of significance (e.g., vehicles, sports memorabilia, coins, furniture): _____

Personal debts (e.g., credit cards, mortgages, loans): _____

Balance owing on each debt: _____

Additional contacts (e.g., financial planner, lawyer, pharmacist): _____

5. HOME SAFETY CHECKLIST

If your mother or father is not fully ready for institutionalized care, one option may be for her or him to remain at home. For your loved one's safety, comfort, and ease of mobility around the home, you will have to realistically evaluate his or her home then make some adjustments. You may also have to carefully evaluate your parent's abilities to remain independent at home. In no specific order, here are a few recommendations:

☐ Place nonskid mats inside and outside of a shower or bath-tub.

☐ Mount grab bars on the walls around the shower, bathtub, and toilet.

☐ Install a smoke alarm (closer to the bedroom is preferable); check and replace the batteries regularly.

☐ Purchase a home fire extinguisher. Keep this in a central spot (e.g., your parent's kitchen) and check this regularly to ensure proper operation.

☐ Replace or install new lighting to brighten up darker rooms and hallways (a lighter or brighter tone of paint can also be very effective).

☐ Remove throw rugs from the floor.

☐ Secure or remove loose carpeting.

☐ Replace patterned carpeting (which may be confusing to older eyes).

☐ Provide extra phones (e.g., having one phone in the kitchen and another in the bedroom, gives a senior more accessible choices, when needed).

☐ De-clutter the surroundings. Remove unneeded furniture and create an open path for walking or wheelchair use.

☐ Replace doorknobs with handle levers for ease of opening.

☐ Replace water faucet taps with handle levers for ease of operation.

☐ Move dishes and glasses to lower shelves to reduce unnecessary reaching.

☐ Replace dishes and glasses with plastic products to reduce accidental breakage, if dropped.

- ☐ Consider installing a stair lift to ease access to upper and lower floors.
- ☐ Paint the tops of steps a lighter colour (or choose a brighter tone of carpeting) to provide better visibility.
- ☐ Place a list of family and emergency phone numbers conspicuously by the telephone.
- ☐ Replace a full-sized vacuum cleaner with a built-in system (reduces the need to lug a heavy machine around the home).
- ☐ Tighten loose stair railings.
- ☐ Install a wheelchair ramp, if necessary, outside of the home.
- ☐ Clean out the refrigerator or pantry on a regular basis. Dispose of spoiled food (note that even canned foods have a "best before" date for safe consumption).
- ☐ Transfer cereals or grains from boxes to sealed plastic containers for safer storage.
- ☐ Tuck any extension cords safely behind furniture rather than stretch them across an open floor. This will reduce the risk of tripping.
- ☐ Hire a reputable housekeeper to assist with cleaning.

6. RESEARCHING LONG-TERM CARE FACILITIES

Photocopy this page and bring it with you as you tour the facilities. Rate each point on a scale of one to five (with one being "poor" and five being "excellent") and make any additional notes on the reverse side of the sheet. If you are viewing numerous facilities, keep your comparison worksheets together.

Care Centre Information

Facility name:
Facility address:
Date visited:
Contact name:
Building appearance:
Building condition and upkeep:
Location:
Parking:
Greeting:
Cleanliness:
Lighting:
Resident transferability within property:
Additional services (e.g., hair care, physiotherapy, nail care):
Staff and resident interaction:
Resident-to-resident interaction:
Room size:
Room shape:
Room location:
Food and food service:
Dietary requests:
Cost for care:
Date of last building inspection:
Date of last elevator inspection:
Emergency evacuation:
Emergency lighting:

Religious denomination:
Resident activities:
Staff experience:
Medication lock-up:
Visiting restrictions:
First impressions:
Comments heard from others:
***Note Any Further Comments below.**

7. DRIVING SAFETY CHECKLIST

Is your aging parent still driving a vehicle? If so, you have every right to be concerned. It's up to you to carefully evaluate your loved one's abilities and urge him or her to hand over the keys when driving becomes too risky.

Answering the questions below will provide you a time line as to when this becomes necessary:

1. Does your parent have reduced reaction time behind the wheel?
2. Has your parent been recently involved in an increased number of accidents (even minor fender-benders)?
3. Does your parent rely less on shoulder checking for other motorists?
4. Does your parent ignore using the vehicle's turn signals?
5. Does your parent drive too slowly or quickly for traffic conditions?
6. Has your parent recently received an increased number of traffic violation tickets?
7. Does your parent stubbornly insist that he or she is "just fine" with driving and blame other drivers for their apparent mistakes?
8. Does your parent try to turn the ignition on or off while the car remains in gear?
9. Has your parent ever mistaken the accelerator pedal for the brake pedal or vice versa?
10. Does your parent ever get lost while driving (on very familiar routes)?
11. Does your parent misjudge distances, such as between cars or when stopping for traffic lights?
12. Has your parent ever driven through a red light or stop sign without noticing it?
13. Does your parent appear more nervous behind the wheel?
14. Does your parent tire more easily when driving?

If you have answered "Yes" to the majority of these questions, it is time to approach your parent (or have a doctor do this instead) to recommend parking the car permanently. Doing so is for the safety of your parent, other motorists, pedestrians, and you.

8. MEDICAL HISTORY LOG

Similar to the Caregiver's Document Worksheet, copies of this important information should also be distributed amongst siblings.

Health-care card number: _____

Family doctor's name: _____
Family doctor's clinic name: _____
Family doctor's clinic address: _____
Family doctor's clinic phone number: _____

Pharmacist's name: _____
Pharmacy address: _____
Pharmacy phone number: _____

Current medical condition(s): _____
Blood type: _____
Family health issues: _____
Allergies: _____

Previous major operations: _____
Dates of operations: _____
Injuries: _____
Date of most recent complete physical exam: _____

Date of most recent dental work: _____
Reason for most recent dental work: _____
Dentist's name: _____
Dentist's address: _____
Dentist's phone number: _____

Alternate treatments sought (e.g., massage, Reiki): _____

Peculiar symptoms noted and dates: _____

_____
_____
_____
_____
_____

9. MEDICATION LOG

With this worksheet, you can record and track your parent's medication history. Pay careful attention to dosages, side effects, and responses. This information will be very useful to doctors and care staff you may encounter. Should you have any questions, consult with your doctor or seek a second medical opinion.

Name of medication: _____

Prescribing doctor: _____

Date of prescription: _____

Dosage: _____

Reason for prescription: _____

New or ongoing prescription? _____

Dosage increases and decreases: _____

Special instructions (e.g., take with food): _____

Side effects: _____

Responses (is medication effective or ineffective?): _____

_____

Name of medication: _____

Prescribing doctor: _____

Date of prescription: _____

Dosage: _____

Reason for prescription: _____

New or ongoing prescription? _____

Dosage increases and decreases: _____

Special instructions (e.g., take with food): _____

Side effects: _____

Responses (is medication effective or ineffective?): _____

_____

Name of medication: _____

Prescribing doctor: _____

Date of prescription: _____

Dosage: _____

Reason for prescription: _____

New or ongoing prescription? _____

Dosage increases and decreases: _____

Special instructions (e.g., take with food): _____

Side effects: _____

Responses (is medication effective or ineffective?): _____

_____

10. CAREGIVER'S FINANCIAL EXPENSES LOG

If you are acting as your parent's trustee, you will be required to complete and submit extensive financial spreadsheets, noting all expenses made. Using the following table, note any specifics of either one-time or ongoing expenses. Remember to keep sales receipts and copies of your parent's bank statements for your records.

Date	Amount Spent	Store Name	Reason for Expense